QUALITY IMPROVEMENT IN HEALTHCARE

Sara Miller McCune founded SAGE Publishing in 1965 to support the dissemination of usable knowledge and educate a global community. SAGE publishes more than 1000 journals and over 800 new books each year, spanning a wide range of subject areas. Our growing selection of library products includes archives, data, case studies and video. SAGE remains majority owned by our founder and after her lifetime will become owned by a charitable trust that secures the company's continued independence.

Los Angeles | London | New Delhi | Singapore | Washington DC | Melbourne

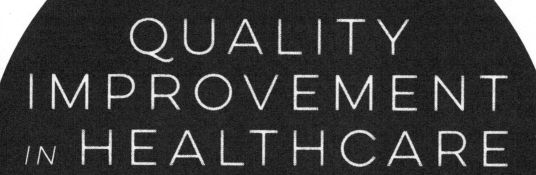

QUALITY
IMPROVEMENT
IN HEALTHCARE

A GUIDE FOR STUDENTS
AND PRACTITIONERS

MARIA KORDOWICZ
A. NIROSHAN SIRIWARDENA

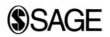

Los Angeles | London | New Delhi
Singapore | Washington DC | Melbourne

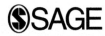

Los Angeles | London | New Delhi
Singapore | Washington DC | Melbourne

SAGE Publications Ltd
1 Oliver's Yard
55 City Road
London EC1Y 1SP

SAGE Publications Inc.
2455 Teller Road
Thousand Oaks, California 91320

SAGE Publications India Pvt Ltd
Unit No 323-333, Third Floor, F-Block
International Trade Tower, Nehru Place
New Delhi 110 019

SAGE Publications Asia-Pacific Pte Ltd
3 Church Street
#10-04 Samsung Hub
Singapore 049483

Editorial Arrangement © Maria Kordowicz and A. Niroshan Siriwardena, 2023

Editor: Laura Walmsley
Assistant Editor: Sahar Jamfar
Production Editor: Neelu Sahu
Copyeditor: Elaine Leek
Proofreader: Rosemary Campbell
Indexer: Michael Allerton
Marketing Manager: Ruslana Khatagova
Cover Design: Sheila Tong
Typeset by KnowledgeWorks Global Ltd
Printed in the UK

Library of Congress Control Number: 2022945547

British Library Cataloguing in Publication data

A catalogue record for this book is available from the British Library

ISBN 978-1-5297-6261-7
ISBN 978-1-5297-6260-0 (pbk)

At SAGE we take sustainability seriously. Most of our products are printed in the UK using responsibly sourced papers and boards. When we print overseas we ensure sustainable papers are used as measured by the PREPS grading system. We undertake an annual audit to monitor our sustainability.

Dedications

Maria Kordowicz: To my mama, Anna Rollason, for nurturing my scholarship, and to Professor Mark Ashworth, my PhD supervisor, mentor and friend.

Aloysius Niroshan Siriwardena: To my wife, Caroline, and daughters, Ishani and Elanor, for always being a source of strength, support and inspiration, to Davis Balestracci who initially fired my enthusiasm for improvement and to my many teachers, colleagues and students whom I continue to learn from.

Contents

About the Authors

Dr Maria Kordowicz BSc(Hons) MSc MRES PhD ProfCertHSCMGT PGCE HE FHEA CMBE AFBPSS MIHM FCMI PPABP CPSYCHOL FRSA

Maria is Associate Professor in Organisational Behaviour and Director of the Centre for Interprofessional Education and Learning at the Faculty of Medicine and Health Sciences at the University of Nottingham. Maria is a Chartered Psychologist in research and teaching and a Coaching Psychologist. She is presently a Trainee Person-Centred and Experiential Psychotherapist at the Sherwood Psychotherapy Training Institute. Maria has had an almost 20-year career in the health and social care sector, holding several senior leadership positions and advisory roles in a range of settings. She directs the qualitative research, evaluation and team development consultancy ResPeo. Maria is an affiliate academic at King's College London, Lincoln, London Southbank and Birmingham Universities, leading and advising on health services research and evaluation. Her interests lie in understanding healthcare organisations, predominantly utilising qualitative ethnographic methods. She sits on a number of research and evaluation boards nationally and internationally, most recently looking at the impact of AI on the healthcare workforce. Maria co-develops the mental health outcome measure PSYCHLOPS, which has been used by the World Health Organization and Médecins Sans Frontières. Maria's PhD from King's College London explored quality improvement in primary care ethnographically.

Aloysius Niroshan Siriwardena MBBS MMedSci PhD FRCGP

Niroshan (Niro) Siriwardena is Professor of Primary and Prehospital Health Care at the University of Lincoln. He is director of the Community and Health Research Unit at the University of Lincoln, a research centre which focuses on quality improvement and implementation research, including studies aimed at development and evaluation of quality measures and health technologies in primary care and ambulance services. He is also director of Lincoln Clinical Trials Unit and an Honorary Professor at Cardiff University. He trained in medicine at St Bartholomew's Hospital Medical College, London and in general practice in Lincolnshire, followed by research training at Nottingham and De Montfort Universities. He has published over 150 research papers in leading journals including the *BMJ*, *Lancet*, *Vaccine*, *Stroke*, and *Sleep*, supported by funding from the National Institute for Health and Care Research, Research Councils UK, the Health Foundation and the Wellcome Trust.

Acknowledgements

Past and current staff of the Community and Health Research Unit at the University of Lincoln.

SECTION A

INTRODUCING QUALITY IMPROVEMENT

1

INTRODUCTION

THE IMPORTANCE OF QUALITY AND IMPROVEMENT

Quality of healthcare was not much talked about when medicine was taught before the turn of the century, but nowadays quality and quality improvement are central to thinking in health, whether by policymakers, clinicians or administrators.

This was because it was generally assumed that healthcare was a good thing, imbued with positive attributes, people and outcomes, whereas the reality is, of course, quite different. We know, from many major reports and inquiries in the UK and elsewhere, that harms from healthcare are all too common (Department of Health, 2000; Institute of Medicine (US), Committee on Quality of Health Care in America, 2001). Healthcare improvement has been affected by the same assumption, that it was necessarily a good thing, but a poorly thought-out quality improvement initiative can also just as easily do harm.

Previous surveys have suggested that quality improvement is poorly understood by many clinical and non-clinical health and social care staff (Apekey et al., 2011; Phung et al., 2016) so this book aims to provide an accessible text for health and social care practitioners and managers.

ABOUT US

We have both worked in the field of quality improvement for many years, which all told amounts to over five decades between us. During this time we have worked as improvement scientists in various capacities, including as clinicians, managers, and academics. We have worked in organisations, large and small, including local general practices, countywide, and regional and national healthcare organisations, where we have had an opportunity to lead and collaborate on projects from small-scale to national in scope. Our relationship with quality improvement has been one that recognises the messy and complex nature of health and social care. Our interests, experience and learning in quality improvement at these various levels led to conversations about quality improvement and to the development of ideas for this textbook. As experts in quality improvement in healthcare, both as practitioners and academics, we have drawn on our practice and research in writing this book, upholding the principle of the person-centred approach to quality improvement. We have also taken a critical and questioning approach to the subject of improvement rather than producing a generic improvement guide and have adopted different approaches, whether psychological, sociological or theoretical, to the topic.

WHY WE WROTE THIS BOOK

Quality improvement is at the forefront of thinking for all healthcare professionals. As we go about our work as healthcare practitioners and managers, in whatever setting we happen to be in, most of us see a myriad of opportunities to improve what we are doing, how we are doing it and the results and experience we achieve for those using the service. This is not only triggered by concerns or complaints from patients and service users but our own feeling as healthcare practitioners or managers that things could be better.

We wanted to write an accessible 'go to' textbook for clinicians and healthcare professionals studying, designing and implementing quality improvement, taking into account advances in research and thinking in this area. The book seeks to straddle both the academic and practical domains of quality improvement in healthcare, and will act as a key reference text for academics, clinicians and healthcare managers alike.

This book explores healthcare quality improvement from multiple perspectives. We outline a range of models and toolkits used in the field. Crucially, the book underlines the need for rigorous evaluation in quality improvement and presents established and emerging evaluation methods in this area. Furthermore, readers are encouraged to self-reflect on their roles as improvers, and to design interventions with sustainability in mind.

WHY YOU SHOULD READ THIS BOOK

This book is aimed at both novice audiences as a learning companion and more experienced quality improvement practitioners as a reference volume. Readers are encouraged to look at quality improvement from different disciplinary perspectives, whilst appraising and analysing opportunities and pitfalls of quality improvement in healthcare. Throughout the book we have focused on the English healthcare context for case studies and examples, but comparative examples have been drawn upon, to ensure the text is relevant to international audiences. We also hope that we have remained cognisant of the English policy context, and prompt the reader to remain reflective of the socio-political context within which they operate.

NAVIGATING THE BOOK

The textbook is organised into four sections (A–D), each containing chapters ordered in such a way as to build on learning, and develop depth of knowledge, if the reader reads the chapters in order. However, each chapter is written as free-standing, written in a practical way to engage the reader from the outset, and intended to enable the reader to refer to these separately, while being able to see links to other relevant sections.

The introductory section (Section A) serves to give an overview of the text and key terms, and provide a rationale for the book itself, as well as for quality improvement in healthcare. The definition of quality in health is highly contested and therefore poses challenges for quality improvement approaches; notably, notions of quality range from the socially constructed to the tangible and therefore measurable. These chapters set the scene.

Following the introduction (Chapter 1), we highlight key concepts and definitions (Chapter 2), which will be revisited and expanded in later chapters. 'Why improve quality?' (Chapter 3) defines quality and its domains, covers concepts such as improvement, and explains why improvement has become so important in the context of potential harms, variation and consumerism. It describes some of the structures and mechanisms by which healthcare organisations have sought to bring about improvement, such as clinical governance and regulation and the importance of an ethical approach to improvement.

The second section of the book focuses on the multiple perspectives (Section B) surrounding the concept and practice of quality improvement in healthcare. It enables the reader to gain insights into the interplay of the policy context (Chapter 4); quality improvement in health over time will be explored, as well as its impact on health organisation and resourcing and how quality improvement is approached 'in the field'. Patient safety (Chapter 5) is presented as a crucial driver of quality improvement. A range of key theoretical perspectives (Chapter 6), including sociological, psychological, health economic and interdisciplinary, are unpicked, helping to shape readers into multidisciplinary scholars and practitioners.

The third section covers different approaches, models and toolkits for improvement (Section C). It presents the established and newer or emerging methods, in the academic and operational literature, illustrating these with case studies and exercises, to enable readers to apply these ideas to their areas of interest. We discuss how to identify problems (troubleshooting), and understand and analyse processes (operationalising quality improvement) using a range of qualitative, quantitative and visual techniques (Chapter 7). The chapter discusses why theories, models and frameworks are important for planning improvement and developing solutions for solving problems. Different methods including clinical audit, the model for improvement and plan–do–study–act, are explained, ending with a discussion of more complex approaches such as Lean and Six Sigma. In looking at working with others (Chapter 8) we cover issues of leadership, patient and user involvement and coaching for improvement.

The final section on evaluating improvement (Section D) provides readers with the knowledge necessary to be able to evaluate and monitor the effectiveness and efficiency of their improvement work, through a range of approaches. In 'How to evaluate quality improvement?' (Chapter 9) we cover the concept of logic models and programme theories, and go on to describe various experimental, quasi-experimental, mixed methods and embedded evaluative designs. Self-evaluation (Chapter 10) is an important but often neglected aspect of improvement, which is about encouraging self-reflection and learning to bring about improvement and insight in oneself. Finally, sustainability (Chapter 11) is not just about sustaining and spreading improvement by translating successful improvement to different contexts, but is also about working in a way that is environmentally aware and sustainable in today's society.

REFERENCES

Apekey, T. A., McSorley, G., Tilling, M. and Siriwardena A. N. (2011) Room for improvement? Leadership, innovation culture and uptake of quality improvement methods in general practice. *Journal of Evaluation in Clinical Practice*, 17: 311–18.

Department of Health (2000) *An Organisation with a Memory: Report of an Expert Group on Learning from Adverse Events in the NHS*. London: The Stationery Office.

Institute of Medicine (U.S.), Committee on Quality of Health Care in America (2001) *Crossing the Quality Chasm: A New Health System for the 21st Century*. Washington, DC: National Academy Press.

Phung, V. H., Essam, N., Asghar, Z., Spaight, A. and Siriwardena, A. N. (2016) Exploration of contextual factors in a successful quality improvement collaborative in English ambulance services: cross-sectional survey. *Journal of Evaluation in Clinical Practice*, 22: 77–85.

2

KEY CONCEPTS AND DEFINITIONS

Chapter summary

This chapter will define key concepts in quality improvement. These will be expanded upon and provide a glossary which will lay the foundations for later chapters.

QUALITY

Quality of healthcare: 'the degree to which health care services for individuals and populations increase the likelihood of desired health outcomes and are consistent with current professional knowledge' (Institute of Medicine (U.S.), Committee on Quality of Health Care in America, 2001).

Quality domains: structure, process and outcome (Donabedian, 1966).

Quality outcomes: patient safety, patient experience and clinical (or cost) effectiveness (Darzi, 2008).

Patient experience: whether or not certain processes or events occurred during a particular visit, a specific episode of care, or over a specified period (Coulter et al., 2009).

Patient satisfaction: patient ratings of their care using categories for better or worse care.

Logic model: a visual representation of the problem, population and priorities or aims, together with inputs, and participants and activities leading to outputs and outcomes for improvement (Siriwardena and Gillam, 2013).

Programme theory: a detailed description of how and why an intervention could or should work and the relationship between the intervention inputs (activities and participants) and outcomes in relation to the context in which they are implemented (Siriwardena and Gillam, 2013).

Clinical governance: a system through which NHS organisations are accountable for continuously improving the quality of their services and safeguarding high standards of care by creating an environment in which excellence in clinical care will flourish (NHS Executive 1998).

Regulation: any set of influences or rules exterior to the practice or administration of medical care that imposes rules of behaviour (Brennan and Berwick, 1996).

Principlism: an ethical framework which includes doing good (beneficence), not doing harm (non-maleficence), creating autonomy, and being fair to all (equity or distributive justice) (Beauchamp and Childress, 2019).

POLICY

Policy: a written down set of principles to help guide behaviours and decisions.

White Paper: UK government guidance on a complex issue setting out proposals for future legislation.

Audit: an inspection of information held about a particular service, for instance to gauge its performance.

Quality and Outcomes Framework (QOF): pay-for-performance scheme for UK general practice where practices are remunerated for meeting pre-established quality targets.

Care Quality Commission (CQC): the independent regulator of all health and social care services in England.

Purchaser–provider split: a service delivery model in which third-party payers or commissioners are kept organisationally separate from service providers.

Quality Indicator: standardised, evidence-based measure of healthcare quality.

Arm's-length body (ALB): a public body with a role set out in law and with a degree of autonomy from the Secretary of State which plays an important role in supporting the health and care system. ALBs include organisations of varying size and degrees of independence from government, from small advisory committees with no independent budget to large organisations employing thousands of public servants and administering billions of pounds of public money.

New Public Management: an approach to improve efficiency of public service using private sector management models such as incentives.

Department of Health and Social Care: UK governmental body responsible for national health policy, led by the Secretary of State for Health and Social Care.

Discourse: the identification and description of the spoken and written word including communications, conversation, or a formal discussion of a subject.

PATIENT SAFETY

Patient safety: freedom for a patient from unnecessary harm or potential harm associated with health care (Council of the European Union, 2009) or the reduction of risk of unnecessary harm associated with healthcare to an acceptable minimum (WHO, 2010).

Safety culture: organisational values and actions related to patient safety.

Patient safety incident: an event or circumstance that could have resulted, or did result, in unnecessary harm to a patient.

Patient safety incident type: incidents that share common features related to administration, prevention, diagnosis or a clinical process, procedure or treatment or a combination of these.

Patient safety outcome: the effect the incident has, either in part or in whole, on the patient, and can include the type of harm, its severity or its physical, psychological, social or economic impact.

Root cause analysis (RCA): a technique for structured risk identification and management which seeks to understand the how and why an error occurred and how it might be prevented.

Significant event audit or analysis (SEA): systematic and detailed analysis of individual cases in which there has been a significant occurrence (not necessarily involving an undesirable outcome for the patient) to ascertain what can be learnt about the overall quality of care and to indicate changes that might lead to future improvements (Pringle, 2000).

Incident or safety reporting system: a way of recording and categorising patient safety to provide accountability to stakeholders, communicate with other professionals, respond to patients and families, monitoring risk within organisations and providing learning to prevent future incidents (WHO, 2020).

TROUBLESHOOTING

Process mapping: a method of seeking to understand, with those involved, the detail of how healthcare is provided, including what happens, when and how, and who receives or does not receive care, as well as how it achieves its effects.

Model for improvement: a model summarising what an improvement initiative is trying to accomplish, how it will be known that change is an improvement and what change can be made that will result in an improvement.

Clinical audit: a systematic activity that involves measuring performance for one or more predefined criteria, each against a standard, and repeating this until the standard is attained or until a new standard is set.

Audit criterion: explicit statement that defines what element of care is being measured.

Audit standard: the level of care to be achieved for an audit criterion.

Plan–do–study–act (PDSA) cycle: an approach to rapid experimentation designed to develop, test and implement change (Gillam and Siriwardena, 2013).

Lean management or **Lean:** an integrated sociotechnical system whose main objective is to eliminate waste by concurrently reducing or minimizing supplier, customer, and internal variability (Rotter et al., 2019).

Six Sigma: the goal of reducing defects or errors to less than six standard deviations which means fewer than 3.4 defects per million (Chassin, 1998).

WORKING WITH OTHERS

Communication: the conveying or exchanging of information by a range of media. Effective communication is concerned with how accurately the information being conveyed is received and understood.

Organisational culture: the ideas, rituals, social behaviours and customs of an organisation.

Team: a group of people with complementary skills, usually grouped together to complete a job, task or project.

Stakeholder: someone who has a direct or indirect interest in an organisation or project.

Organisational development: the theory and practice of techniques that influence organisation change, usually with the aim of progressing organisational functioning.

EVALUATION

Evaluation: aim to assess the effectiveness (relative to a comparator), impacts (change in organisational structures, process or patient outcomes), or success (relative to goals or a logic model) of a quality improvement intervention (Danz et al., 2010).

Statistical process control: a set of graphical and statistical techniques for analysing data over time, understanding whether a process is in control and showing common cause (natural, random) variation or whether it is exhibiting unexpected or special cause variation (unnatural, non-random).

PICO: patient (or population), intervention, comparator and outcome.

RCT: randomised controlled trial in which an intervention is assessed against one or more randomly assigned comparators reducing the chance of confounding and some types of bias.

Complex intervention: an intervention with more than one, and usually several, interacting components.

Cluster randomisation: randomisation of a clinician or organisational unit delivering the intervention to a group or cluster of patients.

Blinding: the treatment or comparator is disguised so that neither the patient nor the clinician knows which has been given.

Bias: a systematic error introduced at any phase of research, including study design, data collection, data analysis or publication.

Confounding: a confounder (confounding variable or factor) is a variable that influences both dependent variable and independent variable causing a spurious and alternative explanation for an association.

Ethnography: an approach to understanding people and cultures within their context, usually through observation.

Non-randomised design: an uncontrolled (before-and-after), non-randomised and quasi-experimental (non-randomised control group, interrupted time series, non-randomised stepped wedge) design.

Interrupted time series (ITS): a design that analyses a change in the rate of change of a measurement over time before or after an intervention takes place.

Process evaluation: a qualitative or mixed methods approach used to understand the detail of the intervention, how and why the change occurred, and whether the same change could occur elsewhere if it was introduced in the same way elsewhere.

Embedded design: a design characterised by adaptive improvement and internal evaluation programmes which interact with each other during the process of improvement and evaluation so that both co-evolve and adapt as they learn from each other.

SUSTAINABILITY

Sustainability: the extent to which goods or services can be sustained.

Scale and spread: refers to the roll-out of an intervention at a larger scale and through replication in other contexts.

Degrowth: a school of thought concerned with the shrinking rather than growing of economies, typically in order to reduce the strain on resources and for environmental sustainability.

REFERENCES

Beauchamp, T. L. and Childress, J. F. (2019) *Principles of Biomedical Ethics*, 8th ed. New York: Oxford University Press.

Brennan, T. A. and Berwick, D. M. (1996) *New Rules: Regulation, Markets, and the Quality of American Health Care*. San Francisco: Jossey-Bass Publishers.

Chassin, M. R. (1998) Is health care ready for Six Sigma quality? *Milbank Quarterly*, 76 (4): 565–91, 510.

Coulter, A., Fitzpatrick, R. and Cornwell, J. (2009) *The Point of Care. Measures of Patients' Experience in Hospital: Purpose, Methods and Uses*. London: The King's Fund.

Council of the European Union. *European Council (2009) Recommendation on patient safety, including the prevention and control of healthcare associated infections*. Brussels, Belgium. Available at: https://www.consilium.europa.eu/uedocs/cms_Data/docs/pressdata/en/lsa/108381.pdf [accessed 24.1.23)

Danz, M. S., Rubenstein, L. V., Hempel, S., Foy, R., Suttorp, M., Farmer, M. M. and Shekelle, P. G. (2010) Identifying quality improvement intervention evaluations: is consensus achievable? *Quality and Safety in Health Care*, 19 (4): 279–83.

Darzi, A. (2008) *High quality care for all. NHS Next Stage Review final report*. London: Department of Health and Social Care. Retrieved from www.gov.uk/government/publications/high-quality-care-for-all-nhs-next-stage-review-final-report.

Donabedian, A. (1966) Evaluating the quality of medical care. *Milbank Memorial Fund Quarterly*, 44 (3): Suppl:166–206.

Gillam, S. and Siriwardena, A. N. (2013) Frameworks for improvement: clinical audit, the plan-do-study-act cycle and significant event audit. *Quality in Primary Care*, 21 (2): 123–30.

Institute of Medicine (U.S.), Committee on Quality of Health Care in America (2001) *Crossing the Quality Chasm: A New Health System for the 21st Century*. Washington, DC: National Academy Press.

NHS Executive (1998) *A first class service*. London: Department of Health.

Pringle, M. (2000) Significant event auditing. *Scandinavian Journal of Primary Health Care*, 18 (4): 200–2.

Rotter, T., Plishka, C., Lawal, A., Harrison, L., Sari, N., Goodridge, D., Flynn, R., Chan J. and Kinsman, L. (2019) What is lean management in health care? Development of an operational definition for a Cochrane Systematic Review. *Evaluation and the Health Professions*, 42 (3): 366–90.

Siriwardena, A. N. and Gillam, S. (2013) Understanding processes and how to improve them. *Quality in Primary Care*, 21 (3): 179–85.

World Health Organization & WHO Patient Safety (2010) *Conceptual framework for the international classification for patient safety version 1.1: final technical report January 2009*. World Health Organization. Retrieved from https://apps.who.int/iris/handle/10665/70882

WHO (World Health Organization) (2020) *Patient safety incident reporting and learning systems: technical report and guidance*. Retrieved from www.who.int/publications-detail-redirect/9789240010338.

3

WHY IMPROVE QUALITY?

Chapter summary

This chapter discusses the meaning of quality and its growing importance for patients, professionals and commissioners, in the context of changing relationships between the public and health professions, the choice agenda, clinical governance and regulation. It ends with considerations of regulatory and ethical issues related to quality improvement.

Summary and learning points

- Understanding quality
- Defining quality, its domains and elements
- Harms from healthcare
- Reducing variation
- Improving quality and reducing harm
- Changing relationships between the public and professionals
- Better information and choice for the public, payers and professionals
- Clinical governance: quality and accountability
- The role of regulation
- The ethics of quality improvement

UNDERSTANDING QUALITY

The notion of quality, central to thinking in today's health services, is still a contested idea. Part of the difficulty with the idea of quality is that it is relative, in that it is the 'standard or something as measured against other things of a similar kind' (Oxford English Dictionary). Quality is also relative to the person judging it, which although this judgement might be relative to expectations and compared with something, it also depends on their perspective. The Institute of Medicine defined quality as 'the degree to which healthcare services for individuals and populations increase the likelihood of desired health outcomes and are consistent with current professional knowledge' (Institute of Medicine (U.S.), Committee on Quality of Health Care in America, 2001). In this definition, the word 'desired' can also be considered as being relative to the perspectives of different individuals or populations and as being judged against alternative healthcare services.

Clinicians might see quality in terms of what things are there to support care (including premises or guidelines), what they are doing (for example, the extent to which guidelines are being followed), or what effect they are having (such as whether patients get better), whereas patients and service users will also reflect on the results of their care but also their experiences of it, and funders will additionally consider value for money. In reality, all of these perspectives will be relevant to all stakeholders, but to different degrees. The judgements will be based on different priorities, comparisons and expectations rooted in the personal experience and knowledge of each.

The importance of improving quality of care and providing safe care is central to the core values of all healthcare professions and professionals. Its origins go back to the ideas of putting patients first and doing no harm, as stated in the Hippocratic Oath, which were revised in the 1960s, of which key tenets still permeate modern professional guidance (Walton and Kerridge, 2014).

The pressure to focus on quality has increased with the changing relationship between medicine, health services, patients and users, but the nature of what quality means has changed from one that is clinician-centred to one that puts patients first and adopts a greater balance between patient, clinician and wider stakeholder perspectives of quality.

The changing relationship between healthcare providers and consumers has also been driven by availability of information, including the wider reporting of health service failures, increased knowledge about potential for harm from doctors (iatrogenesis) and other clinicians, and a greater awareness of the enormous variation in healthcare and outcomes, the so-called postcode lottery of care.

Individual and system failures, harm and variation have also driven developments which promote individual and corporate responsibility for improvement through clinical governance and regulation and these ideas are being incorporated into health service curricula.

DEFINING QUALITY

Although ideas of quality and quality improvement are contested, a number of essential concepts have been proposed and refined through several influential reports and papers. The key ideas are neatly summarised by Allen-Duck and colleagues in their review of quality concepts, based on searching general and medical dictionaries, public domain websites and academic databases, which defined healthcare quality as 'the assessment and provision of effective and safe care, reflected in a culture of excellence, resulting in the attainment of optimal or desired health' (Allen-Duck et al., 2017). The texts cited below are by no means comprehensive but help to develop an understanding of the, often confusingly expressed, terminology of quality.

Avedis Donabedian in a seminal paper developed the concept of the three quality *domains* of structure, process and outcome, which have helped greatly to further the understanding of quality (Donabedian, 1966). 'Structure' refers to what is there to support care, including premises, facilities, drugs, equipment, funding, protocols and guidelines. 'Process' describes what is being done and encompasses all the activities that go into providing healthcare, from direct clinical care to other important actions supporting this, from healthcare management to cleaning. 'Outcome' describes what effect the structures and processes have on patients and includes traditional clinical measures such as survival (or mortality), lengths of hospital stay and costs but also encompasses patient-reported outcome and experience measures. Donabedian stated: 'As I have repeatedly said: structure–process–outcome is a servant, not a master. I never intended to build my reputation on this paradigm. I only offered it as a handy classification scheme. I know that it has deeper meaning …' (Harteloh, 2003).

The Institute of Medicine (IOM), in their widely cited report *Crossing the Quality Chasm* (Institute of Medicine (U.S.), Committee on Quality of Health Care in America, 2001), proposed a number of quality *elements*, including safety, timeliness, effectiveness, efficiency, equity, patient-centredness, as key elements of quality (usefully recalled by the mnemonic STEEEP). The first five of these are widely understood. 'Safety' describes care that does not result in harm. 'Effectiveness' links care to evidence of positive outcomes. 'Efficiency' encompasses cost-effectiveness and value for money. 'Equity' describes care that is provided fairly to patients of different (including protected) characteristics. The last, patient-centredness, although widely used, is a highly disputed and fuzzy concept (Siriwardena and Norfolk, 2007), even among experts (Scholl et al., 2014a). A systematic review of the literature, for example identified 15 inter-related dimensions of patient-centredness, which were then combined into an integrative model of the concept (Scholl et al., 2014b).

Darzi in his Next Stage Review distilled the *outcomes* of care into the triad of patient safety, patient experience and clinical effectiveness (Darzi, 2008). While each is an important and independent area of quality outcomes, they are in fact related. A systematic review found that measurements of safety, experience and effectiveness, although measuring different aspects of the quality triad are usually correlated with each other (Doyle et al., 2013). Cost-effectiveness or productivity is also referred to in the report, so the third outcome of the Darzi triad might be better regarded as clinical (and cost) effectiveness, where cost-effectiveness and productivity relate closely to efficiency.

Patient satisfaction is often confused with patient experience. Although both can use surveys or questionnaires, satisfaction is more challenging to interpret from a quality and measurement perspective. Patient satisfaction involves patients rating their care using categories for better or worse care. It is problematic for quality assessment or measurement because it is a multidimensional concept in which a patient's rating of their experience is influenced by their expectations (Delnoij, 2009). For example, if a patient is used to and expects a particular type of consultation with their doctor, they might be very satisfied with it, even if they did not receive aspects of care they value and feel themselves, on reflection, to be important.

Patient experience, on the other hand, is less affected by expectation because patients are asked to report 'whether or not certain processes or events occurred during a particular visit, a specific episode of care, or over a specified period' (Coulter et al., 2009). Such processes or events could be either positive or negative from a patient's perspective.

Both satisfaction and experience rely on a person's memory of the event, satisfaction on the memory of how they felt and experience on what actually occurred. Patient experience is therefore a better measure than satisfaction from a quality (improvement) perspective because it reduces the problem of 'overly positive responses' due to patients' low expectations or their tendency to avoid negatively rating clinicians (Ahmed et al., 2014; Burt et al., 2018). This latter bias partly explains why clinician ratings of satisfaction tend to be high, even when patient experience might be less favourable.

If patient experience is considered to also incorporate timeliness and patient-centredness, we can see that the IOM and Darzi elements of quality map reasonably well onto each other. The Donabedian domains and Darzi elements of quality can be combined and presented in a matrix which allows us to describe health-related technologies, activities and measures in terms of safety, experience or effectiveness and as structures, processes or outcomes (see Table 3.1 for an example).

Table 3.1 Quality domains and elements for a surgical operation (hip replacement)

Elements	Domains		
	Structure	**Process**	**Outcome**
Patient safety	e.g. Surgical checklist	e.g. Aseptic technique	e.g. Infection
Patient experience	e.g. Theatre or ward	e.g. Preoperative assessment	e.g. Patient reported outcome or experience
Clinical (cost-) effectiveness	e.g. Artificial hip	e.g. Joint replacement	e.g. Return to function

HARMS FROM HEALTHCARE

When training in medicine, a teacher used to ask his students, 'What is the greatest cause of death and disease in the community?' The answer he wanted from us was not heart disease or cancer, but doctors and drugs. This was an important lesson from the writings of Ivan Illich, who popularised the idea of iatrogenesis in the 1970s (Illich, 1977).

In his magnum opus *Medical Nemesis* (Illich, 1977), Illich described and decried not only direct harms from doctors and drugs, so-called clinical iatro-genesis, but also social iatrogenesis, the medicalisation of non-illness, and cultural iatrogenesis, in which medical expertise was expropriating areas of normal life such as birth, child-rearing and death. Although, the origins of 'first do no harm' or *'primum non nocere'* are debated, the importance of patient safety is more relevant today than ever, as harms and failures from use of drugs and treatments in hospital or by community practitioners increases with the widening cadres and capabilities of medical and non-medical professionals.

There is a large and expanding literature documenting adverse events in hospital and community settings, whether due to diagnostic error (Gunderson et al., 2020; Kostopoulou et al., 2008), medication (Assiri et al., 2018; Laatikainen et al., 2017), procedures (de Vries et al., 2008) or being at risk in the care setting (Long et al., 2013). In hospital, adverse events are estimated to affect 1 in 10 patients, of which over two-fifths are considered to be preventable, almost half lead to disability, and 1 in 13 to death (de Vries et al., 2008).

Unfortunately, high profile health service failures and ensuing inquiries have been needed to provide a stimulus for measures to strengthen systems of quality and safety. Notable examples include the Kennedy Inquiry (Kennedy, 2001) following the Bristol Royal Infirmary scandal where deaths in children undergoing cardiac surgery were unusually high, and the Francis Report into the failings at the Mid Staffordshire NHS Foundation Trust (Inquiry, 2010; Inquiry, 2013). These and others and have highlighted tragic shortfalls in the quality of care, communication, culture and leadership, and fundamentally exposed the failure that resulted from not putting patients first and not listening to them or those who spoke on their behalf.

REDUCING VARIATION

The expansion in health information has revealed the huge variation in modes of delivery, costs of provision and health outcomes that exist. The lack of a positive relationship between provision, costs and outcomes implies that a great deal of variation is unwarranted and due to provider-induced demand rather than public need (Wennberg et al., 1982).

Indeed, there is much published evidence to suggest that those at greatest need of healthcare are those least able to access it, the so-called 'inverse care law'. This concept was first proposed by Julian Tudor Hart, who wrote that 'The availability of good medical care tends to vary inversely with the need for it in the population served. This inverse care law operates more completely where medical care is most exposed to market forces, and less so where such exposure is reduced' (Hart, 1971).

Sources of variation in healthcare are many and varied but can be summarised in terms of inputs, the two main inputs being patients or healthcare provision and its measurement. Patient variation is also termed case-mix, where people may be different in their attributes (e.g. age, sex, socioeconomic deprivation) but also in the types of conditions and severity of illness that they present with. Provider variation includes the type of health or care staff, the policies or guidelines they work to, the health technologies (including equipment or drugs) they apply, the processes they work to and the way that measures are produced. The inputs can be expanded, either as a whole or in specific areas to form a 'cause and effect' (sometimes called a fishbone or Ishikawa) diagram (Figure 3.1).

Each of these may be influenced by other factors (represented by the subsidiary arrows). All the inputs may vary and interact to affect outcomes of effectiveness and cost-effectiveness, safety and experience in different ways. Improvement seeks first to reduce variation by introducing standardised, consistent and reliable inputs, including adjusting these for case-mix, where this might be a source of variation, before then trying strategies to improve the process.

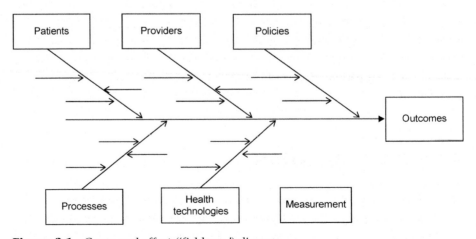

Figure 3.1   Cause and effect ('fishbone') diagram

IMPROVING QUALITY AND REDUCING HARM

Although improving quality and reducing harm is often complex, not straightforward and non-linear, a good way to understand what we are trying to improve and how this might be done is through a simple logic model (Figure 3.2).

A logic model first describes the problem we are seeking to address, the population we are focused on helping, and the improvement aims or priorities (3Ps). Then it considers the various inputs, including any factors depicted in the cause-and-effect diagram above. The logic model next describes those participants who will engage in the quality improvement initiative and what activities they will undertake to improve the outcome(s) of interest.

In the immediate or very short term this is designed to lead to outputs which can be measured in some way, either quantitatively or qualitatively. Finally, a positive quality improvement initiative will lead to improved outcomes, which can also be measured, in the short, medium and long term.

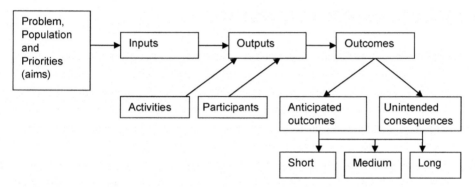

Figure 3.2 A general logic model for improvement

Importantly, for a logic model to make sense, and this is often forgotten, there needs to be a rationale, usually described as programme theory, which explains how and why the participant activities will lead to improvements in outputs and outcomes. Sometimes, despite the best intentions, a quality improvement initiative leads to unintended adverse effects. Sometimes these cannot be predicted, but often with careful thought beforehand they can be foreseen and prevented.

BETTER INFORMATION AND CHOICE

Before and since the Bristol Royal Infirmary scandal there have been efforts to increase publicly available information to patients, families and professionals to help them select services on the basis of quality. The agenda of 'choice' was developed in the 1990s in the United States (Enthoven and Kronick, 1989a, 1989b), advanced through initiatives such as the Patient's Charter, made explicit in the Next Stage Review (Darzi, 2008) and embodied as a principle in England's NHS constitution (Department of Health, 2015). The policy background is described in further detail in Chapter 4.

Despite the rhetoric of choice as a driver of quality, there is very limited evidence that public reporting of performance data changes patient behaviour or improves care (Metcalfe et al., 2018). In their systematic review of 12 randomised or quasi-experimental studies of the effects of public health performance data, Metcalfe and colleagues (Metcalfe et al., 2018) included data from over 7500 providers and over 3 million patients in the US, Canada, Korea, China and the Netherlands, which showed only low-certainty evidence that public release of performance data had limited effects on long-term healthcare use by patients or providers or affected provider performance. The review also showed low-certainty evidence that public release of performance data may slightly improve some patient outcomes, and one study suggested it may have differential effects on disadvantaged populations.

CHANGING RELATIONSHIPS

The publicity around health service failures, greater access to information and cultural change over the past half century have contributed to a transformation in the relationship between health services, practitioners, patients and the public. This transformation has led to expectations of greater openness and transparency from clinicians and providers, in direct communication but also in the quality and quantity of information provided about individual care and the quality of care being provided more generally.

In line with clinician–patient communication being more patient-centred and a greater understanding of what this means in practice, there is an expectation that information is provided about the quality of services and outcomes of care. This has been partly driven by notions of choice, expanding the market of providers, and devolving commissioning closer to patients, who are encouraged to choose services based on information about services.

Unfortunately, marketisation has also brought with it the related ideas of performance and performance-related pay, which has led to commodification of patients and other unintended adverse consequences (Gillam and Siriwardena, 2010; Gillam et al., 2012).

CLINICAL GOVERNANCE

Clinical governance was introduced at the dawn of the 50th anniversary of the NHS in the UK government White Paper *The New NHS*, as 'a system through which NHS organisations are accountable for continuously improving the quality of their services and safeguarding high standards of care by creating an environment in which excellence in clinical care will flourish' (Department of Health, 1997).

It was introduced together with other innovations including the National Institute for Clinical Excellence (NICE, the forerunner to the current National Institute for Health and Care Excellence), the Commission for Healthcare Excellence (now the Care Quality Commission) and the National Service Frameworks. Although the emphasis was on quality and quality improvement, in the areas of effectiveness, efficiency, patient safety and satisfaction (Scally and Donaldson, 1998), and some early documents referring to seven pillars of clinical governance (clinical effectiveness, risk management, patient experience and involvement, audit, staff management, continuing education and training, and information), the key to understanding clinical governance is the link between quality and accountability: in its purest sense it means accountability for quality of care.

This stems back to the criticism highlighted in the Kennedy Report (Kennedy, 2001) of the failure by medical leadership at the Bristol Royal Infirmary to demonstrate accountability and take action in light of the failings of the paediatric cardiac surgeons at the hospital. Sanctions were meted out to the chief executive together with the surgeons by the General Medical Council. Accountability for quality means that chief executives, medical directors and clinicians bear responsibility for the quality of clinical care they, others in the organisation and the organisation as a whole provide to patients. No longer can senior managers claim, as they did in the Bristol case, that quality of care was the responsibility of individual clinicians.

Unfortunately, by making clinical governance more complicated and vaguer than it needed to be, it has been roundly criticised from the outset for polysemy and ambiguity (Goodman, 1998).

ROLE OF REGULATION

Regulation was defined by Brennan as 'any set of influences or rules exterior to the practice or administration of medical care that imposes rules of behaviour' (Brennan and Berwick, 1996). Professional bodies such as the General Medical Council, are responsible for ensuring individual professional standards, while health regulators, for example the Care Quality Commission, are accountable for monitoring and assuring the quality and safety of organisations and national bodies markets, and government or its agents are responsible for controlling the market in health services (Gillam and Siriwardena, 2014).

Brennan and Berwick identified possible ways that regulation might improve care by: detecting and correcting problems; taking action when substandard individuals or organisations are found; spreading exemplars of good practice; encouraging continuous quality improvement; and supporting creativity (Brennan and Berwick, 1996).

In the UK the regulator sets out to monitor, inspect and regulate services to ensure organisations meet fundamental standards of quality and safety, publish inspection findings and performance ratings to inform care choices, and act where the standards are not met.

ETHICS OF QUALITY IMPROVEMENT

On the face of it, quality improvement might be perceived as ethical in itself. Using principlism as an ethical framework one could argue that improving quality is to do good (beneficence), enhancing safety seeks to do no harm (non-maleficence), increasing patient autonomy improves patient experience, and that reducing variation as part of quality improvement efforts augments equity or distributive justice (Beauchamp and Childress, 2019).

A deeper analysis reveals that this simplistic approach leaves many questions unanswered. Cribb and colleagues argue that quality improvement is 'a set of techniques or a "technology"' (Cribb et al., 2020) designed to bring about improvement and, like any other technology, has the potential in the context of a real-life setting to provide no actual benefit, or even to cause harm through unintended adverse effects, to fail to respect patients' rights to autonomy or privacy or be inequitable in its effects (Cribb et al., 2020).

Therefore, it is essential when considering quality improvement initiatives to think carefully about the ethical imperatives of such activities. It will be important to ensure that autonomy is preserved or enhanced by considering issues of consent, confidentiality and information governance as appropriate. The positive effects of interventions need to be maintained by ensuring that there is an evidence base, that their fidelity is preserved, and that any implementation processes are designed to maximise or increase benefits. Potential harms, due to unintended adverse consequences need to be thought about in advance and mitigated as far as possible. Finally, we need to consider whether a quality improvement initiative, inadvertently favours one group of patients compared to another, and consider undertaking a quality impact assessment to understand and mitigate any differential effects.

REFERENCES

Ahmed, F., Burt, J. and Roland, M. (2014) Measuring patient experience: concepts and methods. *Patient*, 7: 235–41.

Allen-Duck, A., Robinson, J. C. and Stewart, M. W. (2017) Healthcare quality: a concept analysis. *Nursing Forum*, 52: 377–386.

Assiri, G. A., Shebl, N. A., Mahmoud, M. A., Aloudah, N., Grant, E., Aljadhey, H. and Sheikh, A. (2018) What is the epidemiology of medication errors, error-related adverse events and risk factors for errors in adults managed in community care contexts? A systematic review of the international literature. *BMJ Open*, 8: e019101.

Beauchamp, T. L. and Childress, J. F. (2019) *Principles of Biomedical Ethics.* New York: Oxford University Press.

Brennan, T. A. and Berwick, D. M. (1996) *New Rules: Regulation, Markets, and the Quality of American Health Care.* San Francisco: Jossey-Bass Publishers.

Burt, J., Abel, G., Elmore, N., Newbould, J., Davey, A., Llanwarne, N., Maramba, I., Paddison, C., Benson, J., Silverman, J., Elliott, M. N., Campbell, J. and Roland, M. (2018) Rating communication in GP consultations: the association between ratings made by patients and trained clinical raters. *Medical Care Research and Review*, 75: 201–18.

Coulter, A., Fitzpatrick, R. and Cornwell, J. (2009) *The Point of Care. Measures of Patients' Experience in Hospital: Purpose, Methods and Uses.* London: The King's Fund.

Cribb, A., Entwistle, V. and Mitchell, P. (2020) What does 'quality' add? Towards an ethics of healthcare improvement. *Journal of Medical Ethics*, 46: 118–12.

Darzi, A. (2008) *High quality care for all. NHS Next Stage Review final report.* London: Department of Health and Social Care. Retrieved from www.gov.uk/government/publications/high-quality-care-for-all-nhs-next-stage-review-final-report.

De Vries, E. N., Ramrattan, M. A., Smorenburg, S. M., Gouma, D. J. and Boermeester, M. A. (2008) The incidence and nature of in-hospital adverse events: a systematic review. *Quality and Safety in Health Care*, 17: 216–23.

Delnoij, D. M. (2009) Measuring patient experiences in Europe: what can we learn from the experiences in the USA and England? *European Journal of Public Health*, 19: 354–6.

Department of Health (1997) *The New NHS.* London: The Stationery Office.

Department of Health (2015) *The NHS Constitution.* London: The Stationery Office.

Donabedian, A. (1966) Evaluating the quality of medical care. *Milbank Memorial Fund Quarterly*, 44 (3): Suppl:166–206.

Doyle, C., Lennox, L. and Bell, D. (2013) A systematic review of evidence on the links between patient experience and clinical safety and effectiveness. *BMJ Open*, 3 (1).

Enthoven, A. and Kronick, R. (1989a) A consumer-choice health plan for the 1990s. Universal health insurance in a system designed to promote quality and economy (1). *New England Journal of Medicine*, 320: 29–37.

Enthoven, A. and Kronick, R. (1989b) A consumer-choice health plan for the 1990s. Universal health insurance in a system designed to promote quality and economy (2). *New England Journal of Medicine*, 320: 94–101.

Gillam, S. and Siriwardena, A. N. (2010) *The Quality and Outcomes Framework: QOF – Transforming General Practice.* Oxford: Radcliffe Publishing.

Gillam, S. and Siriwardena, A. N. (2014) Evidence-based healthcare and quality improvement. *Quality in Primary Care*, 22: 125–32.

Gillam, S. J., Siriwardena, A. N. and Steel, N. (2012) Pay-for-performance in the United Kingdom: impact of the quality and outcomes framework: a systematic review. *Annals of Family Medicine*, 10: 461–8.

Goodman, N. W. (1998) Clinical governance. *BMJ*, 317: 1725–7.

Gunderson, C. G., Bilan, V. P., Holleck, J. L., Nickerson, P., Cherry, B. M., Chui, P., Bastian, L. A., Grimshaw, A. A. and Rodwin, B. A. (2020) Prevalence of harmful diagnostic errors in hospitalised adults: a systematic review and meta-analysis. *BMJ Quality and Safety*, 29 (12): 1008–18.

Hart, J. T. (1971) The inverse care law. *Lancet*, 1: 405–12.

Harteloh, P. P. (2003) The meaning of quality in health care: a conceptual analysis. *Health Care Analysis*, 11: 259–67.

Illich, I. (1977) *Limits to Medicine. Medical Nemesis: The Expropriation of Health* (new ed.). Harmondsworth and New York: Penguin.

Inquiry (2010) *Independent Inquiry into care provided by Mid Staffordshire NHS Foundation Trust, January 2005 – March 2009* (the Francis Report). 2 vols. London: The Stationery Office.

Inquiry (2013) *Report of the Mid Staffordshire NHS Foundation Trust Public Inquiry: Executive summary.* London: The Stationery Office.

Institute of Medicine (U.S.), Committee on Quality of Health Care in America (2001) *Crossing the Quality Chasm: A New Health System for the 21st Century.* Washington, DC: National Academy Press.

Kennedy, I. (2001) *Learning from Bristol: The report of the Public Inquiry into children's heart surgery at the Bristol Royal Infirmary 1984–1995.* London: The Stationery Office.

Kostopoulou, O., Delaney, B. C. and Munro, C. W. (2008) Diagnostic difficulty and error in primary care – a systematic review. *Family Practice*, 25: 400–13.

Laatikainen, O., Miettunen, J., Sneck, S., Lehtiniemi, H., Tenhunen, O. and Turpeinen, M. (2017) The prevalence of medication-related adverse events in inpatients – a systematic review and meta-analysis. *European Journal of Clinical Pharmacology*, 73: 1539–49.

Long, S. J., Brown, K. F., Ames, D. and Vincent, C. (2013) What is known about adverse events in older medical hospital inpatients? A systematic review of the literature. *International Journal for Quality in Health Care*, 25: 542–54.

Metcalfe, D., Rios Diaz, A. J., Olufajo, O. A., Massa, M. S., Ketelaar, N. A., Flottorp, S. A. and Perry, D. C. (2018) Impact of public release of performance data on the behaviour of healthcare consumers and providers. *Cochrane Database of Systematic Reviews*, 9: CD004538.

Scally, G. and Donaldson, L. J. (1998) Clinical governance and the drive for quality improvement in the new NHS in England. *BMJ*, 317, 61–5.

Scholl, I., Zill, J. M., Harter, M. and Dirmaier, J. (2014a) How do health services researchers understand the concept of patient-centeredness? Results from an expert survey. *Patient Preference and Adherence*, 8: 1153–60.

Scholl, I., Zill, J. M., Harter, M. and Dirmaier, J. (2014b) An integrative model of patient-centeredness – a systematic review and concept analysis. *PloS One*, 9: E107828.

Siriwardena, A. N. and Norfolk, T. (2007) The enigma of patient centredness, the therapeutic relationship and outcomes of the clinical encounter. *Quality in Primary Care*, 15: 1–4.

Walton, M. and Kerridge, I. (2014) Do no harm: is it time to rethink the Hippocratic Oath? *Medical Education*, 48: 17–27.

Wennberg, J. E., Barnes, B. A. and Zubkoff, M. (1982) Professional uncertainty and the problem of supplier-induced demand. *Social Science and Medicine*, 16: 811–24.

SECTION B

PERSPECTIVES

4

THE POLICY CONTEXT

━━ **Chapter summary** ━━━━━━━━━━━━━━━━━━━━━━━━━━━━━━━

This chapter will outline the policy background to quality improvement in the health service in England over time. It will become clear that performance capture for the purpose of quality improvement has become ubiquitous within the NHS and the public sector. A key learning point of this chapter is how closely interwoven policy narratives and mandates are with how quality is conceptualised and enacted within the NHS.

━━ **Summary and learning points** ━━━━━━━━━━━━━━━━━━━━━━━

- What is policy?
- Quality in policy since the foundation of the NHS to the present day
- What is a White Paper?
- What is audit?
- How are policies made?
- What is QOF?
- What is discourse?
- The role of NHS management and quality
- New Public Management and quality
- Features of New Public Management
- Introducing Michel Foucault
- Concluding remarks

What is policy?

A policy is typically a written down set of principles to help guide behaviours and decisions. Policies are a statement of intent, setting out expectations and are enacted through organisational procedures. Policies are usually adopted officially.

Within the health services, policies can be made at the local level, often reflecting national government policy. There is a web of organisations working at the micro, meso and macro levels of the healthcare system in England, each with their own sets of policy and guidance. Policies are made to influence organisations and behaviour at one, some or all of those three levels.

The governmental body responsible for national health policy is the Department of Health and Social Care, led by the Secretary of State for Health and Social Care.

QUALITY IN POLICY SINCE THE FOUNDATION OF THE NHS TO THE PRESENT DAY

Since the foundation of the NHS in a post-World War II climate in 1948, government policy papers revealed financial tensions and power shifts between the clinical and managerial. As early as two years into its operations, a ceiling on NHS expenditure was imposed and successive reports highlighted the need for financial astuteness, such as the Guillebaud (1956) and Porritt (1962) reports. The financial pressures on the NHS have continued to mount over consecutive decades, with significant austerity cuts in spending imposed under the Conservative/Liberal Coalition government of 2010 and embraced by the Conservative government of 2015 onwards at the time of writing. Improving quality is often justified through its cost-effectiveness to the taxpayer and can therefore be in part seen as the attempt to do more with less resource. In this vein, providers of NHS services bid for contracts and their success rests on being able to demonstrate not only their capacity to provide quality services, but also to do this at lower costs than its competitors.

It was Margaret Thatcher's reforms that played a key role in establishing the management of quality within the health service and the public sector more broadly. The 1980–1990 decade brought an unrelenting focus on efficiency, resource control and accountability. Under Thatcher, the introduction of competitive tendering for ancillary NHS services demanded that potential providers be able to demonstrate a level of both financial and service performance which would secure contracts. Towards the end of Thatcher's time in office, internal markets, along with a purchaser/provider split, were introduced into the NHS, working on the assumption that increased competition drives service performance. Thatcher commissioned the Griffiths Report (1983), led controversially by Sir Roy Griffiths, the former Deputy

Chairman of Sainsbury plc. This era is often seen as heralding managerialism in the NHS, through the introduction of market disciplines into policy. The perceived lack of service quality was identified by Griffiths to sit with the lack of obvious leadership in the NHS. In this vein, he is famously cited as stating:

> if Florence Nightingale were carrying her lamp through the corridors of the NHS today she would almost certainly be searching for the people in charge.

Moving into John Major's government (1990–1997), 'The Patient's Charter' (Department of Health, 1991) recognised the central role of patient choice in improving service quality. Policy discourse of the patient as a consumer was introduced, whereby more options should be offered to the patient to enable them to 'vote with their feet'. Considerations about best value to the taxpayer were highlighted and it was proposed that the patient voice should be at the centre of service and policy decisions. In order for this to happen, patients had to be well informed and there were calls for greater transparency about NHS service performance, through publicly available performance data, e.g. hospital league tables. However, some of the limitations of measuring performance against top-down indicators as a marker of quality came to the fore in 1996, when league tables were criticised by professional bodies as pointless and misleading after ranking some of the country's leading hospitals among the worst performers (Goldstein and Spiegelhalter, 1996).

Since the inception of The Patient's Charter, incorporating service user views into quality service provision does demonstrate a greater awareness of the 'beholder's' perspective. It could be argued that traditionally quality was seen largely in patriarchal terms as, for example, in the definition: 'degree to which the care delivered is in agreement with medical professional criteria' (Simons and van Mansvelt, 1976). Today, the patient voice challenges this traditional patriarchal view and has more prominence in policy design (e.g. by taking on board responses to national patient surveys) and service delivery (e.g. through patient participation groups).

There was a clear assumption within policy that through treating patients more like consumers, services would 'compete' for satisfied clientele and therefore would drive up their quality standards in order to achieve this. However, this assumption was not without its flaws, as the following rules of consumerism indicate. Seldom are the unwell in a position to make a full choice about where and how they are treated, and health service provision largely remains tied to the locality in which a patient lives or works.

For consumerism to take effect:

- Alternatives need to exist
- Moving from one option to another should be practically possible (Barnes and Walker, 1996: 58)

Another notable development under John Major was the National Health Service and Community Care Act 1990 – partnerships to ensure quality of care in the community. It is important to note that there is a difference between an Act and a policy. A policy is a plan, which may not involve specific laws, whereas an Act is a legislative process. As we know, policies outline a course of action, however there is little that can be done to enforce them. Acts are enforceable laws. This Act was a seminal event in the health and social care quality landscape – it introduced an internal market into the supply of healthcare in the United Kingdom, making the state a facilitator rather than a supplier of health and social care provision. Arguably, this cemented the evaluation of quality on competitive market-based criteria, namely value for money and consumer demand.

A further aim of the Act was to ensure that adults aged 18 years or over who were eligible for services had the right to a full assessment of their needs and the services provided were to be individually tailored to meet the needs identified. An element of tailored care included consideration being paid to those who could be treated in the community rather than within in- and outpatient settings. This gave rise to a propagation of 'care in the community', whereby the government promoted a policy of deinstitutionalisation, so that where possible those requiring physical and mental health care would be treated in their homes rather than in a statutory setting. Whilst considered more humane and person-centred to treat patients in the home, an overriding aim of the policy was to generate cost savings by caring for people in a less expensive setting. This dehospitalisation wave of reforms was also supported by developments in pharmacological treatments of serious mental illness. Some key criticisms of the implementation of the 'care in the community' approaches included inadequate resourcing to support vulnerable members of society outside of inpatient settings, the overburdening of untrained family members with complex care for their loved ones, and the closure of institutional premises without the creation of new community settings in parallel.

The National Health Service and Community Care Act therefore brought with it a complexity around how quality of care is enacted in statutory versus the home setting and the desirability of both from the perspective of the service users and their carers. Nonetheless, these reforms continued to be veiled in the rhetoric of client centredness and the consumerist imperative as offering both value for money and greater patient empowerment.

The notion of consumerism as a driver of quality endured under Tony Blair's Labour government (1997–2007). Patient views were now collectively referred to as the 'User Voice', somewhat short-sightedly assuming that all patients speak in agreement with one another and have similar notions of what quality of care means to them. Blair's 'New' Labour also wholeheartedly embraced the Thatcherian principles of driving quality improvement through performance management. The policy language of the time in the 'Modernising Government'

(Department of Health, 1999a) and 'Saving Lives: Our Healthier Nation' (Department of Health, 1999b) White Papers became increasingly influenced by private sector principles. The focus was on reviewing NHS services and identifying best suppliers for them. New targets and performance indicators were introduced to achieve 'real improvements' and 'quality and effectiveness'. These goals were supported by a new information technology strategy and infrastructure, regular audits and data submission from those on the ground to management and, in turn, to the government bureaucrats.

What is a White Paper?

Governmental White Papers give guidance on complex issues. They also set out the government's proposals for future legislation. Typically, incoming governments use White Papers to set out their vision for their term in office.

What is an Audit?

Taken from the language of financial accounting, an audit in health indicates an inspection of information held about a particular service for instance to gauge its performance.

It is worth noting, that this top-down target-driven audit-led era of governance is coined 'New Public Management' (Ferlie et al., 1996), with its origins firmly rooted in Thatcherite principles of public sector management. The features and subsequent impact of New Public Management on the control of the public healthcare sector will be explored in more depth later in this chapter.

How are policies made?

There is a plethora of stages of policy-making models in the literature. They tend to focus on the following stages (adapted from Howlett et al., 2003):

Setting the agenda – what is of importance and to whom?
Policy formulation – exploring options, bringing the policy document together.
Decision-making about adoption – the government decides whether or not to adopt the policy.
Implementation – putting the policy into practice and making changes in line with the policy.
Evaluation – has the policy had the desired effects? Were there any unexpected or spinoff consequences? How can the policy be improved?

It can be argued that the policy-making process is more complex than a linear staged model suggests. Instead, the stages may well overlap and be revisited at different points in the process, rendering the policy-making process one of changeable and, at times volatile, flow. Further, we can think of the process as cyclical, with the findings of the evaluation feeding back into the stages of policy-making.

Under New Labour, targets were designed to be 'tougher but attainable' and there was a recognition of the need to focus on priority areas. Contracts were put into place between central government and local services, with local providers having to evidence the quality of their service delivery. There was a particular drive for reducing health inequalities, with a clear focus on primary care for public health gains, in order to reduce the utilisation of more expensive secondary care. 'The NHS Plan' (Department of Health, 2000) paved the way for standard setting with an annual assessment of NHS organisations, along with the publication of results in the public domain. It is within this climate that the Quality and Outcomes Framework (QOF) was introduced in general practice in 2004. You will see QOF used as one of the many illustrative examples of quality improvement schemes throughout this book.

What is QOF?

The Quality and Outcomes Framework, or QOF for short, is a pay-for-performance scheme, whereby general practitioners (GPs) are remunerated for meeting pre-established 'quality' targets.

QOF was introduced in 2004, with a budget of £1.8 billion earmarked for the scheme. Targeted payments directly linked to indicator achievement would be made yearly and indicators revised, to ensure continuous quality improvement.

Prior to the introduction of QOF, GPs were paid for list sizes, the number of doctors within the practice and the number and types of services provided. QOF, at the time presented as a voluntary scheme, was to account for about a third of a practice's income and appeared to be a welcome scheme, offering GPs an opportunity for an earmarked pay rise. In 2003, an overwhelming majority of GPs (79.4%) voted to accept the QOF.

The election of 2010 saw the Conservatives return to power in a coalition government with the Liberal Democrats. Their loftily titled White Paper 'Equity and Excellence: Liberating the NHS' (Department of Health, 2010) set out the plans for GP Commissioning, a reduction in management costs by more than 45% and £20 billion of efficiency savings. Alongside this, the new Health and Social Care Act 2012 focused on greater transparency and accountability, with increased powers given to regulatory bodies, such as the Care Quality Commission (CQC) replacing Primary Care Trusts (PCTs), in order to monitor and inspect health and social care services and take enforcement action where necessary. It was clear that performance management through the use of quality indicators and monitoring was not going anywhere any time soon.

Crucially, under the Coalition government (2010–2015), with David Cameron as Prime Minister, the NHS underwent unprecedented large-scale reform and restructuring. The most notable of these are the wave of changes commonly referred to as the 'Lansley Reforms', named after the Secretary of State for Health from 2010 to 2012, Andrew Lansley, whose department engineered them. The reforms consisted of an overhaul of the management and organisational structure of the NHS, whilst emphasising the markets and internal competition as a driver of quality in the provision of healthcare. Despite the push for quality, the Coalition era saw a dramatic drop in government funding for the NHS, as part of the start of its austerity measures (attempts to reduce government spending in order to control public sector debt). Lansley faced much criticism for the reforms, which were largely viewed as deliberate commercialisation and 'backdoor privatisation' of the NHS.

Indeed, a King's Fund report (2013), highlighted that NHS policy reforms held the goal of improving 'NHS performance and hence the quality of patient care'. This statement highlights a tendency in the academic and policy literature to use the words 'performance' and 'quality' almost interchangeably, indicating that high-quality care is the product of good performance and that a quality health service is also a high-performing one. To take this further, this suggests that performance measures and standard frameworks in healthcare have an overarching aim of achieving high quality care. Furthermore, the King's Fund claimed that the Lansley reforms damaged the NHS stating that 'arguments about privatisation distract from the much more important and damaging impacts of the reforms on how the NHS is organised and the ability of its leaders to deal with rapidly growing financial and service pressures' (2013: xx).

The Lansley reforms were also criticised for creating confusing structures with dispersed or confused lines of accountability. Indeed, during this period, the organisational landscape of healthcare, including the proliferation of health and social care Arm's-length bodies (ALBs) became far more complex and arguably more difficult for a patient to navigate. ALBs are a range of public bodies, including non-ministerial departments, such as NHS England and NHS Improvement (which merged in 2019), responsible for overseeing the use of resources in the NHS in order to support the ministerial Department of Health and Social Care. These bodies also have quality assurance as part of their mandates, focusing on the following elements of quality as defined in statute: safety, clinical effectiveness and patient experience.

> The NHS is organising itself around a single definition of quality: care that is effective, safe and provides as positive an experience as possible. (National Quality Board, 2013)

The next key policy development that scholars of quality improvement should be aware of is the learning and resulting recommendations stemming from the Mid

Staffordshire public inquiry. It is this period which brought about a greater focus on organisational culture as an enabler of, or as in the case of the Mid Staffordshire NHS Foundation Trust, an impediment to, quality. Hundreds of hospital patients died as a result of substandard care and failings at two hospitals in Mid Staffordshire between January 2005 and March 2009. Examples of poor care included patients left in soiled bedding and having to drink water from flower vases as none was provided to them. On the surface Mid Staffordshire was a high-performing Trust, which in 2008 acquired Foundation status, awarded to *hospitals demonstrating the highest clinical standards, quality leadership and an excellent record of patient safety*. This calls into question how quality is measured, recognised and rewarded, given that 'Mid Staffs' is viewed as one of the most shocking modern-day hospital scandals. Indeed, the decisions made in pursuit of Foundation Trust status, in particular cost-cutting exercises, are viewed as a key contributory factor in the persistence of poor-quality care.

The scandal resulted in a 31-month public inquiry chaired by Robert Francis QC. The resulting report (Inquiry, 2010, 2013) highlighted the unacceptably high mortality rates and the abuses of care. This was a full public inquiry into the role of the commissioning, supervisory and regulatory bodies in the monitoring of the Trust. The report made 260 recommendations for learning and improvement, namely in relation to safe staffing levels, openness and transparency, and creating healthier organisational cultures. Crucially, wilful neglect has since become an offence, whereby there is criminal liability where an individual who has the care of another individual by virtue of being a care worker ill-treats or wilfully neglects that individual.

The King's Fund (2013) provides an apt quote here, capturing the impetus resulting from 'Mid Staffs' to move towards improved organisation cultures, an improvement which rest on leadership:

> Leaders at all levels need to develop an understanding of culture and recognise that culture – not regulation, direction, supervision and punishment – is what determines behaviour in NHS trusts. Culture is the way we do things around here; it is the current in the river; the hidden determinant of organisational direction; the manifestation of values. Leaders must then work together to nurture healthy, positive cultures and that will require them to embrace the concept of collective leadership.

The lessons stemming from the inquiry were framed as a push for cultural change by Jeremy Hunt's Department of Health in the report 'Culture change in the NHS: Applying the lessons of the Francis Inquiries' presented to Parliament in 2015.

It is Jeremy Hunt's era as Secretary of State for Health and Social Care (2012–2018) that we look at next. It was not without turbulence. His time in office was marked by the NHS weekend cover debacle and the junior doctors strikes. The former concerned what is viewed as a misinterpretation of a study identifying excess deaths on weekends in NHS settings, which then led Hunt to conclude that there was a Monday to Friday culture in the NHS and that NHS medical consultants needed to regain a sense of vocation to commit more fully to their jobs. This led to much anger amongst medics, which in part was channelled through a social media campaign with weekend work selfies alongside the hashtag #iminworkjeremy. A seven-day NHS plan followed from Hunt, which was widely criticised due to its gaps in workforce planning and funding. Moreover, under Hunt, the Department of Health as it was then known introduced new junior doctors' contracts, with the aim of extending their working hours for which they would not be paid an additional premium. Ninety-eight per cent of British Medical Association (BMA) members voted for strike action, leading to strikes on an unprecedented scale, with junior doctors only providing emergency care. The strike action and resulting negotiations, as well as a High Court challenge, did not go in the favour of junior doctors, with the new contract being implemented through imposition. This era of policy-making is viewed as a time of mistrust and conflict between the government and the medical profession, as well as a reflection of the clash of agendas and understandings surrounding what constitutes sound delivery of quality care.

A final White Paper of note to set the scene for the context in which this book is being written, is the 'Change and Transformation' White Paper. This is a framed by NHS England as a 'call to action', arguing that change needs to happen at a faster rate and become more disruptive. Though change management scholars and practitioners may well know the pitfalls of forcing through change at a fast pace and how it can undermine employee wellbeing, the focus has very much been on continued reform (now more dynamically referred to as 'transformation' in policy discourse) and a recognition of the importance of digital innovation to drive quality. As such, under Secretary of State for Health and Social Care Matt Hancock, we saw the foundation in 2019 of NHSX, which described itself on its former website as 'a joint unit bringing together teams from the Department of Health and Social Care and NHS England and NHS Improvement to drive the digital transformation of care'. Increasingly, quality of care is promoted through the use of smart phone applications for triage and consultations, to achieve cost-savings and great efficiency. Of course, moving to virtual working where possible has been enabled by the challenge of the COVID-19 pandemic. For instance, virtual consultations have been rolled out by GP practices to uphold patient safety, resulting in much discussion as to whether the majority of general practice can be carried out remotely and what the new working model may look like for GPs post pandemic. This unsurprisingly has been met with some opposition, highlighting factors such as the importance of human connection and the impact job design on staff morale and clinical effectiveness.

— What is discourse? —

Discourse in literal terms refers to the identification and description of the spoken and written word. It can therefore refer to communications, conversation, or a formal discussion of a subject. In academic study, discourse refers to the conceptual themes of particular communications. Therefore, when discussing policy discourses, we are interested in the conceptual generalisations conveyed by the policy documents.

THE ROLE OF NHS MANAGEMENT AND QUALITY

In parallel to these developments regarding quality in the NHS, prompted by economic considerations, the debates around clinical versus managerial leadership in the NHS also began almost from the time of the inception of the NHS. Initially, hospitals were clinically led by a matron and a medical superintendent. The Porritt Report (1962) proposed that doctors should hold the position of chief officers of area boards. Four years later, the Farquharson-Lang Report (1966) stated that chief executives need not be medically qualified. The same year, the Salmon Report pushed for raising the profile of the (cheaper) nursing profession in hospital management. The 1970s saw the advent of multidisciplinary management teams and power devolved to local health authorities under the 1972 'NHS Reorganisation' White Paper. It is clear, that there were a number of concerns around the roles managers versus clinicians should play in the administration of the NHS, with managers potentially posing a threat to the clinicians' expertise and the clinicians perhaps not being best utilised or best placed to manage financial resources and lead teams (and paradoxically undermining quality).

As mentioned previously, under Margaret Thatcher's government Sir Roy Griffiths was commissioned to write a report into the effectiveness of the public sector. This appointment was controversial, as Griffiths was a former Deputy Chairman of Sainsbury's supermarkets, a for-profit retail business driven by private sector principles, which were seen to be at odds with the value-driven altruistic public sector ethos (Le Grand, 2003; Le Grand and Bartlett, 1993). In his report (1983) Griffiths emphasised the need for improved management in the NHS.

Thatcher's era of New Public Management brought about increased non-clinical leadership of the NHS, with a power shift away from professionals to budget-holding managers and market incentives to improve efficiency. This continued under New Labour, with numerous commentators lamenting the increased managerialisation of the healthcare sector and the bureaucratic mechanisms employed as methods of control (e.g. McAvoy and Kaner, 1996; Smith, 2001). The shift to Conservative government in the UK somewhat reversed the trend of non-clinical management, with a drive to implement clinical leadership evidenced by GP commissioning, for instance, along with the government's commitment to reduce management costs by almost half. However, the 2020 COVID-19 pandemic context would see Personal Protective Equipment and Track and Trace contracts being awarded 'behind closed doors' to corporate for-profit organisations, highly criticised for their lack of clinical knowledge and clinical leadership, and the resulting lack of quality in service provision.

The next section of this chapter will explore the features of New Public Management in more detail, along with the policy-driven use of incentives to drive quality in the NHS.

NEW PUBLIC MANAGEMENT AND QUALITY

New Public Management is the term that refers to an era of public management based on Thatcherite principles of the introduction of market incentives into the public sector in order to improve efficiency. These principles were embraced by Tony Blair's New Labour government, where performance management regimes became ubiquitous within the public sector. New Public Management also assumes the responsiveness and flexibility of organisations to be able to effectively engage with top-down quality improvement measures. New Public Management is tied to discourses of consumerism, patient voice and choice, and providing best value for the taxpayer. This became a salient feature of competitive tendering where cost was a key determinant in securing contracts to provide NHS services.

Despite adopting a strategic approach to implementing improvements in line with pre-set top-down standards, New Public Management is interesting in the ways through which it proposes to meet its aims. Unlike a traditional Weberian (Weberian refers to the work of Max Weber) bureaucracy structure typically associated with the public sector, namely a formal hierarchical structure and management by rules, New Public Management aims for flexible rather than hierarchical public sector organisations, with management through targets and performance indicators. The goals of New Public Management are supported by an improved information technology infrastructure and increased computerisation to facilitate the collection and monitoring of performance data.

New Public Management signals an indirect rather than direct control (Walsh, 1995). In this vein, it could be argued in line with Carter (1989) that New Public Management created 'decentralisation downwards, not accountability upwards'. Managers retain an ownership over performance indicators, which enables them to practise indirect 'hands off' control. Financial incentives, designed to motivate professionals, are aligned closely to policy goals of increased efficiency and quality.

Another feature of New Public Management is the power shift it brings towards managers and away from older established professional groups, not achieved through direct management, but by surveillance and control from indicator-driven performance management frameworks, of which the primary care pay-for-performance scheme, the Quality and Outcomes Framework (QOF), is an example. This has led some commentators to claim that the traditional professional dominance model (e.g. Freidson, 1970a, 1970b) has been challenged by New Public Management reforms (Ferlie et al., 1996; Hood, 2006). This dynamic has allowed governments to limit the traditional autonomy and power of professionals such as medics, primarily through gaining increased control over their budget decisions. With the introduction of QOF for example, GPs had to justify up to a third of their practice's income on the basis of QOF performance, leading to increased transparency over financial remuneration within general practice, whilst also equating performance success with greater income and vice versa. It could therefore be said that quality became reframed through QOF as something to seek out for external financial gain, rather than as an end in itself.

Whilst QOF was initially introduced as a voluntary scheme, practices were unlikely to opt out of a scheme that would account for up to a third of their annual income. Similarly, the potential stigma attached to being labelled as a 'poor' performer within publicly available league tables also puts a question mark over the voluntary nature of the framework.

New Public Management reforms promote improved performance within healthcare services by offering financial incentives for meeting pre-established quality targets (Ferlie et al., 1996), along with an increase in public transparency, and therefore accountability to the taxpayer. Indeed, a number of studies have demonstrated that the publication of performance data can play a meaningful role in quality improvement (Marshall et al., 2000).

The drive for improving quality in health services through performance indicators can therefore be understood as a product and tool of New Public Management and the introduction of market incentives to improve the efficiency of public services (Walsh, 1995). New Public Management was embraced by New Labour's White Paper 'Saving Lives: Our Healthier Nation' (Department of Health, 1999b) and subsequent policy, with the establishment of targets in priority areas to reduce health inequalities.

However, the 'Health of the Nation' White Paper of the 1992 Conservative government upon which New Labour's 'Our Healthier Nation' was based, was criticised for not promoting evidence-based targets and data capture mechanisms (Department of Health, 1998). Furthermore, a review of the impact of this earlier White Paper suggests that the engagement of GPs with local quality improvement initiatives was slight, and overall GPs lacked an interest in the 'bigger picture' of strategic action nationally. This may be one of the limitations of New Public Management principles, whereby the lack of professional ownership over strategy may result in a sense of isolation from and disengagement from any resulting schemes.

No doubt, New Public Management has paved the way for a culture of increased monitoring and regulation, through the use of electronic surveillance technologies and sanctions in healthcare services, rather than by the direct engagement of clinical professionals. Nonetheless, 'Our Healthier Nation' continued New Public Management discourse with the rhetoric of increased accountability through monitoring and evidence-based target-based quality improvement frameworks. Whilst there is a prominent body of literature arguing that increased managerial interventions undermine clinical professionalism and therefore should be resisted (e.g. Freidson, 1985; Mangin and Toop, 2007), in contrast McDonald, Harrison and Checkland's (2007, 2008) findings point towards the development of a new status quo where surveillance is regarded as legitimate and a necessary tool in quality capture.

It worth noting that the discourse of managerialism became infused with language and quality improvement 'toolkits' of industry. Whilst we shall explore this in more depth later on in the book, the health service has seen a proliferation of industry-based quality improvement mechanisms over the past few decades. A notable example would be Lean, a waste elimination approach in Toyota manufacturing, which has been touted as a panacea for a range of structural ills in the NHS (Radcliffe et al., 2020). Key criticisms of these types of quality management approached are linked to the extent to which they are a 'best fit' within the complex landscape of health and a publicly owned national health service. A feature of several QI toolkits includes the measurement of quality through metrics, creating greater transparency around performance through external information capture, and thus arguably accountability towards the taxpayer. Therefore, the work of the clinician becomes more visible externally, but predominantly through the limited lens of numerical performance capture.

Taking this further, it could be argued that managerialism creates a negative culture of 'bureaucratic accountability', achieved through external surveillance. Clinicians may be critical of this situation but are viewed as demonstrating little resistance to it (Harrison et al., 2002). Increased monitoring poses a further challenge for quality capture. The resulting bureaucracy and a feeling of being 'watched' can lead to clinicians' sense of professionalism being undermined. It is not a new point of view that potentially reducing patient care to a 'pay for reporting' approach can be demotivating and even reduce quality in non-incentivised areas (Kordowicz and Ashworth, 2013).

Following on from this policy trend, that the aforementioned QOF was conceived in 2004 as part of the Department of Health's new General Medical Services Contract (nGMS) and became the dominant model for monitoring the quality of general practice in England on a 'pay-for-performance' basis. Against the policy backdrop of improving the quality of patient care through measurable targets becoming a key preoccupation within health services (Elwyn and Hocking, 2000), QOF became synonymous with general practice quality in the language of health management and policy-makers.

Features of New Public Management

- Indirect rather than direct control (Walsh, 1995)
- Market incentives can improve service efficiency
- Power shift from professionals to managers
- Introduction of targets and performance indicators
- Flexible rather than hierarchical public organisations

INTRODUCING MICHEL FOUCAULT

It is by refining his theory of power, through his studies of the interaction of the state and its subjects, that Michel Foucault developed the notion of governmentality (Foucault in Burchell et al., 1991). Here, he moved away from the traditional understanding of power as lying within the apexes of societal hierarchies. Rather power, as discussed previously, is presented as becoming internalised by professional strongholds through knowledge. According to Foucault, power lies in a loose ensemble of the state and expert groupings, within what he termed a power/knowledge nexus. The medical professional can be viewed in the context of an existing part of this wider nexus, whereby their power is, to an extent, at the mercy of state apparatus.

Thus, the knowledge that professional groups are recognised as experts by the government conversely leads to more effective forms of social control. In Foucault's view, this is because knowledge enables individuals and groups to govern themselves. To apply this to the professions, by recognising certain groups as holding professional power, the government renders them officially capable of enacting government policy. Therefore, the ways in which the professions self-govern are tacitly infiltrated by government influence. Furthermore, knowledge facilitates the creation of self-ruling and auto-regulated groups, resulting in 'the formation of a whole series of specific governmental apparatuses' (Foucault in Burchell et al., 1991).

By applying the Foucauldian lens, we could argue that there is a 'quality agenda' and that this agenda renders clinicians government apparatus. The agenda itself is an example of the enactment of Foucauldian governmentality, whereby it is used to undermine medical power and professionalism in order to grow the reach, influence and power of the state. Though we could argue that quality reforms are often engineered by clinical leaders themselves, rather than solely by government bureaucrats, Foucault would see these leaders as pawns of the government, used as tools to tacitly infiltrate and dismantle the echelons of professional power.

CONCLUDING REMARKS

The purpose of this chapter was for readers to gain a greater understanding of the salient role that government policy and the political landscape play in how quality in health is conceived and enacted. The chapter has provided an overview of key policies since the inception of the NHS which has contributed to the quality agenda and the key public sector discourse surrounding it. It is of note how various stakeholder interests influence how quality is defined and the various linked NHS reforms over time. The problem of defining quality will be explored in the next chapter. We also cannot ignore the economic prerogative and the 'value for money' imperatives which underpin NHS policies and reconfigurations, and the resulting effects that these hold for patients' lived experience of the quality of the care they receive.

Further reading

Ferlie, E., Ashburner. L., Fitzgerald, L. and Pettigrew, A. (1996) *The New Public Management in Action*. Oxford: Oxford University Press.

Stone, D. (2001) *Policy Paradox: The Art of Political Decision Making*. New York: W. W. Norton & Company.

REFERENCES

Barnes, M. and Walker, A. (1996) Consumerism versus empowerment: a principled approach to the involvement of older service users. *Policy and Politics*, 24 (4): 375–93.

Burchell, G., Gordon, C. and Miller, P. (1991) *The Foucault Effect: Studies in Governmentality*. Chicago: University of Chicago Press.

Carter, N. (1989) Performance indicators – backstreet driving or hands off control? *Policy and Politics*, 17 (2): 131–8.

Department of Health (1966). *Farquharson-Lang Report*. London: HMSO.

Department of Health (1996). *Salmon Report*. London. HMSO.

Department of Health (1972) *NHS Reorganisation*. White Paper. London: HMSO.

Department of Health (1991) *The Patient's Charter*. London: HMSO

Department of Health (1992) *The Health of the Nation*. White Paper. London: HMSO.

Department of Health (1998) *The Health of the Nation – A Policy Assessed: Executive Summary*. London: The Stationery Office.

Department of Health (1999a) *Modernising Government*. White Paper. London: The Stationery Office.

Department of Health (1999b). *Our Healthier Nation*. White Paper. London: The Stationery Office.

Department of Health (2000). The NHS Plan. London: The Stationery Office.

Department of Health (2010) *Equity & Excellence: Liberating the NHS*. White Paper. London: The Stationery Office.

Department of Health (2014). *Change and Transformation*. White Paper. London; The Stationery Office.

Elwyn, G. and Hocking, P. (2000) Organisational development in general practice: lessons from practice and professional development plans (PPDPs). *BMC Family Practice*, 1: 2.

Ferlie, E., Ashburner, L., Fitzgerald, L. and Pettigrew, A. (1996) *The New Public Management in Action*. Oxford: Oxford University Press.

Freidson, E. (1970a) *Professional Dominance: The Social Structure of Medical Care*. New Jersey: Transaction Publishers.

Freidson, E. (1970b) *Profession of Medicine: A Study in the Sociology of Applied Knowledge*. New York: Dodd, Mead & Co.

Freidson E. (1985) The reorganisation of the medical profession. *Medical Care Review*, 42: 11–35.

Goldstein, H. and Spiegelhalter, D.J. (1996) League tables and their limitations: statistical issues in comparisons of institutional performance. *Journal of the Royal Statistical Society*, 159 (3): 385–443.

Griffiths, R. (1983) *NHS Management Inquiry*. London: HMSO.

Guillebaud Report (1956) *Report of the Committee of Enquiry into the Cost of the National Health Service*. London: HMSO.

Harrison, S., Dowswell, G. and Milewa, T. (2002) Guest editorial: Public and user 'involvement' in the UK National Health Service. *Health and Social Care in the Community*, 10 (2): 63–6.

Hood, C. (2006) Gaming in targetworld: the targets approach to managing British public services. *Public Administration Review*, 66 (4): 515–21.

Howlett, M., Ramesh, M. and Perl, A. (2003) *Studying Public Policy: Policy Cycles and Policy Subsystems*. Toronto: OUP Canada.

Inquiry (2010) *Independent Inquiry into care provided by Mid Staffordshire NHS Foundation Trust, January 2005 – March 2009* (the Francis Report). 2 vols. London: The Stationery Office.

Inquiry (2013) *Report of the Mid Staffordshire NHS Foundation Trust Public Inquiry: Executive summary*. London: The Stationery Office. [For background to the report and an outline of the government's initial response see https://commonsli brary.parliament.uk/research-briefings/sn06690/.]

King's Fund (2013) Now is the time to transform NHS cultures. Available at: www. kingsfund.org.uk/blog/2013/09/now-time-transform-nhs-cultures.

Kordowicz, M. and Ashworth, M. (2013) Capturing general practice quality – a new paradigm? *British Journal of General Practice*, 63 (611): 288–9.

Le Grand, J. (2003) Part I Theory: Of knights and knaves. In *Motivation, Agency and Public Policy: Of Knights and Knaves, Pawns and Queens*. Oxford: Oxford University Press. pp. 21–3.

Le Grand, J. and Bartlett, W. (eds) (1993) *Quasi-Markets and Social Policy*. London: Macmillan.

Mangin, D. and Toop, L. (2007) The Quality and Outcomes Framework: What have you done to yourselves? *British Journal of General Practice*, 2007; 57 (539): 435–7.

Marshall, M., Shekelle, P. G., Leatherman, S. and Brook, R. (2000) What do we expect to gain from the public release of performance data? A review of the evidence. *JAMA*, 283: 1866–74.

McAvoy, B. and Kaner, E. (1996) General practice postal surveys: a questionnaire too far? *BMJ*, 313: 732.

McDonald, R., Harrison, S., Checkland, K. et al. (2007) Impact of financial incentives on clinical autonomy and internal motivation in primary care: ethnographic study. *BMJ*, 334: 1357.

McDonald, R., Harrison, S. and Checkland, K. (2008) Incentives and control in primary health care: findings from English pay-for-performance case studies. *Journal of Healthcare Organisation & Management*, 22 (1): 48–62.

National Quality Board (2013) *Quality in the New Health System: Maintaining and Improving Quality from April 2013*. London: Department of Health and Social Care.

Porritt, A. (1962) *Review of Medical Services in Great Britain*. London: HMSO.

Radcliffe, E., Kordowicz, M., Mak, C., Shefer, G., Armstrong, D., White, P. and Ashworth, M. (2020) Lean implementation within healthcare: imaging as fertile ground. *Journal of Health Organization and Management*, Oct 14, ahead-of-print. doi: 10.1108/JHOM-02-2020-0050.

Simons, A.J. and van Mansvelt, J. (1976) *Intercollegiale Toetsing in Algemene Ziekenhuizen (Rapport)*. Utrecht: Centraal Begeleidingsorgaan voor de Intercolegiale.

Smith, R. (2001) Editorial: Why are doctors so unhappy? There are probably many causes, some of them deep. *BMJ*, 322 (7294): 1073–4.

Walsh, K. (1995) *Public Services and Market Mechanisms*. London: Macmillan.

5

PATIENT SAFETY

Chapter summary

Patient safety is a key aspect of healthcare quality. It may be a surprise to many people, including those entering a healthcare or related profession or organisation, with the sole intention of doing good and helping others, that healthcare could do just the opposite, and cause harm. The risk of harm increases as the healthcare system increases in complexity, with more organisations and more staff with different areas of expertise, as the numbers of drugs and treatments we can use expand, and as our patients get older and sicker with a myriad of illnesses and possible diagnoses. This has meant, shockingly, that harm from healthcare has become one of the top ten causes of illness and death worldwide according to the WHO (WHO, 2019).

This chapter defines what we mean by patient safety and discusses the types of harm that can arise, it outlines how common and costly patient safety events are, and then considers how we can learn from them to prevent future harms. Prevention involves learning from events, and developing systems for reporting, managing, anticipating and avoiding harm. As in any quality improvement initiative, we need to be able to measure patient safety, so tools for this and measures are discussed. Finally, we describe organisational safety strategies, culture and climate, and explore some of the tools and interventions currently being used in prevention.

Summary and learning points

- Defining patient safety
- Understanding categories of harm
- Incidence, prevalence and costs of harm

- Learning from patient safety events: root cause, critical incident and significant event analysis
- Human factors and systems
- Incident and safety event reporting systems
- Integrated risk management and preventing system failure
- Patient safety measurement tools and measures
- Organisational safety strategies, culture and climate
- Safety tools and interventions: safety checklists, briefings, huddles, walkrounds, handovers and collaboratives

DEFINING PATIENT SAFETY

Quality care, as we have defined it earlier, is care that is effective (and efficient), safe and improves patient experience. As the complexity of healthcare and those who receive it increases, the possibility of unsafe care and harms arising from the provision of healthcare rather than the condition for which it is sought also widen, leading to healthcare-associated harm being one of the top ten reasons for hospitalisation worldwide (WHO, 2019). There are many definitions of patient safety, but put simply it is the 'freedom for a patient from unnecessary harm or potential harm associated with health care' (Council of the European Union, 2009).

A more nuanced definition from the WHO is, 'Patient safety is the reduction of risk of unnecessary harm associated with healthcare to an acceptable minimum. An acceptable minimum refers to the collective notions of given current knowledge, resources available and the context in which care was delivered weighed against the risk of non-treatment or other treatment' (WHO, 2009).

Addressing patient safety has become an increasing concern of policy-makers, researchers, and healthcare professionals, from the concept of iatrogenesis developed by Illich in the 1970s (Illich, 1977) to two seminal reports published 30 years later at the turn of this century, *To Err Is Human* (Kohn et al., 2000) from the Institute of Medicine in the US, and *An Organisation with a Memory* in the UK (Department of Health, 2000).

Both reports and subsequent epidemiological studies of patient safety cite the very high rates of healthcare-associated harms. Around 1 in 10 hospital admissions are associated with a healthcare-associated harm and around half of these are preventable (WHO, 2017).

CATEGORIES OF HARM

The range of potential harms from healthcare is wide and the complexity of types of incident, patient susceptibilities, contributory factors and ways to detect, mitigate, ameliorate or reduce the risk of adverse patient or organisational outcomes has led to complex, internationally agreed taxonomies to describe these (WHO, 2009).

A *patient safety incident* is an event or circumstance that could have resulted, or did result, in unnecessary harm to a patient. *Incident types* describe incidents that share common features, and can be related to administration, prevention, diagnosis or a clinical process, procedure or treatment or a combination of these. *Patient outcomes* are the effect the incident has, either in part or in whole, on the patient and can include the type of harm, its severity or its physical, psychological, social or economic impact. The incident type and patient outcome together can be combined to describe patient safety events (WHO, 2009).

The three commonest patient safety incidents are those related to surgical procedures, medication errors and healthcare-associated infections (WHO, 2017).

━━━━━━━━━━ LEARNING ACTIVITY ━━━━━━━━━━

Harms you have encountered

Think about the commonest types of healthcare-related harms that you have encountered in your practice. What was the harm or incident? How did this affect the patient? How might this have been prevented?

INCIDENCE, PREVALENCE AND COSTS OF PATIENT HARM

Healthcare-associated harm is costly to patients, their families and health services, with estimates amounting to trillions of dollars worldwide. The costs attributable to patient safety events in hospital range from around $3000 to $10,000 per case (in the region of just over £2600 to £8700 at the time of writing) (Mittmann et al., 2012). As well as the costs of death, disability and loss of work for patients and their families, there are the costs of insurance and litigation, together with other hidden costs, such as loss of trust in the system. In contrast, the cost of preventing harm is a fraction of this (Etchells et al., 2012). The incidence and outcome of a patient safety incident varies according to the type of incident and type of setting in which it occurs.

A systematic review of in-hospital adverse events found a median overall incidence of 9%, of which over two-fifths were deemed preventable. Most were due to surgical procedures (two-fifths of cases) or medication-related events (one in six). Although more than half of patients affected experienced no or minor disability, one in 13 patients died as a result (de Vries et al., 2008).

Medication errors are an important source of harm in both community settings and hospitals. A medication error is 'any preventable event that may cause or lead to inappropriate medication use or patient harm, while the medication is in the control of the health care professional, patient, or consumer' (Assiri et al., 2018). Errors can occur anywhere in the process of medication production and delivery, from selection, procurement, storage, ordering and preparing, to dispensing, administration, or monitoring.

Rates of medication error vary according to the studies, setting and error types. Prescribing error rates in community settings range from 2% to 94%, the most common being inappropriate prescribing and monitoring (Assiri et al., 2018). The incidence of preventable adverse drug events (ADEs) has been estimated as 15/1000 person-years, with drug interaction ADEs as 7% and preventable ADEs 0.4% (Assiri et al., 2018). In hospitals, medication errors constitute 7% of medication orders, affecting between a fifth and half of patients admitted and 2 in 100 patient days (Laatikainen et al., 2017; Lewis et al., 2009). Intravenous drug errors are more common, with errors reported in 10% (8–12%) of administrations in the UK, most commonly drugs given at the wrong rate in 3 out of 5 cases or other types of administration errors in almost a third of cases (Sutherland et al., 2020).

LEARNING FROM PATIENT SAFETY EVENTS

When things go wrong, patients and families want open and honest information about what happened, a genuine apology, and a promise that things will improve, with future errors prevented (Sattar et al., 2020). Unfortunately, healthcare practitioners are often slow to respond to errors because they lack training and skills on communicating errors, they fear litigation or blame, or they work in organisations where guidance is unclear or inconsistent, and where there is blame culture or an ethos which is not conducive to disclosure (Sattar et al., 2020). Responding appropriately and learning from errors is vital, and failure to do this has been at the heart of many high-profile failures in healthcare organisations.

There are number of tools such as root cause, significant event or critical incident analysis, which have been used in the past to aid learning from errors and to help to identify ways to prevent these recurring, but it is increasingly recognised that these techniques may themselves be flawed, misapplied or poorly executed, which leads to them failing to improve patient safety (Martin-Delgado et al., 2020).

Root cause analysis is one commonly used range of techniques employed for structured risk identification and management which seeks to understand how and why an error occurred and how it might be prevented. The analysis should be undertaken by a trained team with sufficient time and expertise to question, investigate and explore what happened and why, in an atmosphere of openness and learning which seeks to understand the event from a wide perspective of the system to ensure that changes can avert future similar events from occurring. Several cognitive and physical techniques and instruments have been used in root cause analysis. These include the '5 Whys', a process of repeatedly asking why an event occurred at increasing depth to uncover the root causes. These can be arranged into a causal tree linking the causes and ways that a near miss was avoided or an adverse event could be prevented. Action decision tables can be used to list causes in terms of their potential for harm, the severity of an adverse outcome together with the likelihood of recurrence, as well as the need and method for monitoring, the possibility of detecting future events, and actions to prevent these (Williams, 2001).

Despite widespread use and evidence that root cause analysis can be useful in identifying causes of patient safety events such as interprofessional communication mistakes, human error and problems with healthcare processes, there are problems with the technique conceptually, practically and in terms of its outcomes. A key conceptual problem is that there is often not a single root cause but multiple causes which form a flaw in the system (Vincent, 2004). The focus on single causes means that a system approach is not adequately considered, effective measures are not introduced and the effects are limited or absent (Martin-Delgado et al., 2020). Time or resource constraints, lack of feedback to those who might learn, failure to implement risk controls, and lack of responsibility or accountability for changes (Peerally et al., 2017) together with the use of weak interventions (Kellogg et al., 2017) can also hamper the potential for root cause analysis to be effective.

Another method is critical incident analysis which led to the closely related technique used in primary care of significant event audit or analysis. In significant event audit 'individual cases, in which there has been a significant occurrence (not necessarily involving an undesirable outcome for the patient), are analysed in a systematic and detailed way to ascertain what can be learnt about the overall quality of care and to indicate changes that might lead to future improvements' (Pringle, 2000). Common types of significant event include prescribing errors, failure to action an abnormal result, delayed or wrong diagnoses, failure to refer or deal with an emergency call, breach in confidentiality or a breakdown in communication (Gillam and Siriwardena, 2013). The steps in the audit include identifying events, collecting facts about it, meeting to discuss it, undertaking a structured analysis, monitoring actions and writing up the event. Unfortunately, as in root cause analysis, significant event audit has failed to deliver improvements because of lack of training, poor team dynamics, facilitation or leadership, the emotional demands or poor choice of event (Bowie et al., 2008).

This lack of focus on recommendations, limited effectiveness and the time-consuming nature of root cause analysis or significant event audit, has led to alternative techniques being introduced, such as after-action review (AAR), adverse event debriefing and huddles, SWARM, concise incident analysis (CIA) and investigation of multiple incidents using comprehensive frameworks or multi-incident analysis (Hagley et al., 2019). These alternatives have several features in common, including less time and depth of analysis but a greater attention to the team, communication and systems, as well as focussing on what happened, why, and how it could be prevented in future (Hagley et al., 2019).

Causes of safety events are often multifactorial and due to an interaction between contributing factors, patient characteristics and incident characteristics. Contributing factors are those involved in the development or increased risk of an incident occurring and may be related to staff, patients, the workplace or environment, organisation, or external or other factors.

In most settings and for most incidents there are multiple contributing factors. In hospital settings the commonest adverse events are related to surgical procedures but fewer of these are preventable compared with diagnostic adverse events. In a systematic review, individual human error was found to be the most frequent cause, with system failure causing 3% to 85% (this wide variation being due to differences in data collection methods and classifications used) and equipment failure much less common (Sari et al., 2010).

Learning from incidents can occur at local, institutional, national or international level, referred to respectively as single, double, triple and quadruple loop learning. Single loop learning involves clinicians or managers in localities learning and implementing solutions, whereas double loop learning extends this to managers reviewing clusters of incidents, larger organisational units or institutions, and triple loop learning widens this to national health organisations, regulators, colleges or agencies while quadruple loop learning spreads this internationally (Runciman et al., 2006). For learning at national and international levels, incident and safety event reporting systems are needed to enable a systematic approach to analysis, feedback, learning and improvement.

HUMAN FACTORS AND SYSTEMS

In the preface to the report *To Err Is Human: Building a Safer Health System* the following passage emphasises the importance of systems in making healthcare safer: 'Human beings, in all lines of work, make errors. Errors can be prevented by designing systems that make it hard for people to do the wrong thing and easy for people to do the right thing' (Kohn et al., 2000). In order to design safer systems it is therefore important to have a better understanding of human factors (also termed ergonomics), albeit with the idea of moving away from a person-focused approach to solutions to a system-focused approach (Reason, 2000). Ergonomics is the science of interactions among humans and other elements of a system, and the profession that applies theory, principles, data and methods to design in order to optimise human wellbeing and overall system performance (Dul et al., 2012).

Human error can be categorised into two main types, slips and lapses versus mistakes (Reason, 1995). A slip (external observable) or lapse (internal unobservable loss of memory) is a failure of execution due to deviation from an intended process whereas a mistake occurs when an action is carried out as intended but a failure in planning or problem-solving results in an error. Slips or lapses are usually due to distraction from a routine process and may be caused by a failure of attention, memory, task selection or recognition. Mistakes may be rule-based when good rules are not applied (e.g. not testing for glucose in the urine in someone with weight loss) or applied incorrectly (prescribing aspirin in coronary disease when the patient has a history of allergy) or a bad rule is used (e.g. the misconception that a failed suicide attempt is a 'cry for help' and therefore has a low risk of harm, when the opposite is true). Mistakes can also be knowledge-based when the cognitive demands required to solve a problem are exceeded or subject to bias.

Errors need to be distinguished from violations. Violations are deviations from defined good practice, procedures, standards or rules. They may occur from cutting corners (routine violations), alleviating boredom (optimising violations) or because the problem seems to require an approach outside standard practice (necessary or situational violations.) Violations are more likely to be due to problems with motivation or organisation whereas errors are more likely to be due to lack of information.

Another important distinction is between active and latent errors. The former can lead to instant or early adverse effects, usually occurring in direct care provided by front-line staff, whereas the latter are more likely to lead to a delayed effect and are often due to errors developing more remotely, for example in the management or design of processes.

Reason (2000) developed the Swiss cheese model of error to demonstrate how 'defences, barriers, and safeguards may be penetrated' by a combination of latent and active errors occurring in the context of the system of healthcare. He went on to explain that systems vulnerable to error exhibited the three interacting features of blaming front-line staff, denying the possibility of systemic proneness to error, and a narrow focus on indicators (Reason et al., 2001). He described the condition of 'vulnerable system syndrome' (VSS), present to some extent in all organisations, and amenable to remediation through a process of double loop organisational learning that goes beyond active errors to explore the wider conditions of the system that could lead to error (Reason et al., 2001).

INCIDENT AND SAFETY EVENT REPORTING SYSTEMS

Reporting systems, such as the National Reporting and Learning System (NRLS) in the UK (NPSA, 2004a) and similar systems set up by the Agency for Healthcare Research Quality (AHRQ) in the US, and the Advanced Incident Management

System (AIMS) in Australia (Runciman et al., 2006) are designed to enable patient safety incidents to be recorded and categorised as a means of providing accountability to stakeholders, communicating with other professionals, responding to patients and families, monitoring risk within organisations and providing learning to prevent future incidents (WHO, 2020).

Patient safety incidents can be considered as reportable circumstances, near misses, no-harm incidents, or harmful incidents. A reportable circumstance occurs when a situation arises that has potential for harm, but no incident occurred, for example an expired drug found but never used. A near miss is when an incident occurs but does not get as far as the patient, for example a wrong drug being drawn up, but then not used. No-harm incidents involve patients directly, for example a wrong drug administered, but no harm occurs as a result. Finally, a harmful incident or adverse event is said to occur when, for example, an incorrect dose or use of a drug or procedure results in direct harm to the patient. Harmful incidents can be 'adverse events' which result in preventable harm to a patient or 'adverse reactions' where the harm is not preventable and where the correct processes and procedures were followed (WHO, 2020).

The more serious reportable patient safety events are referred to variously as 'never events', 'serious reportable events', or 'always review and report' incidents but these variations in terminology can be problematic for identifying, comparing, learning from and preventing such occurrences. These are incidents that cause or potentially cause serious harm, are largely preventable, tend to recur, provide potential for significant learning, are identifiable and measurable, and can be included in incident reporting systems (Hegarty et al., 2021). The commonest never events reported in the UK are wrong-site surgery, followed by retained foreign objects and the wrong implant or prosthesis (Omar et al., 2021). Examples of never events in UK general practice generated through a modified Delphi consensus approach are listed in Box 5.1 (de Wet et al., 2014). The most commonly occurring of these, in order of frequency of reporting, were abnormal investigation results not reviewed, prescribing when adverse reaction recorded, and cancer referral not sent (Stocks et al., 2019).

━━━━━━━ LEARNING ACTIVITY ━━━━━━━

Reporting systems

What reporting systems do you use in your organisation? What training have you had to use these? How well do these systems work? How could they be improved?

BOX 5.1   LIST OF NEVER EVENTS IN GENERAL PRACTICE (DE WET ET AL., 2014)

1   Prescribing a drug to a patient that is recorded in the practice system as having previously caused her/him a severe adverse reaction
2   A planned referral of a patient, prompted by clinical suspicion of cancer, is not sent
3   Prescribing a teratogenic drug to a patient known to be pregnant (unless initiated by a clinical specialist)
4   Emergency transport is not discussed or arranged when admitting a patient as an emergency
5   An abnormal investigation result is received but is not reviewed by a clinician
6   Prescribing aspirin for a patient <12 years old (unless recommended by a specialist for specific clinical conditions, for example, Kawasaki's disease)
7   Prescribing systemic oestrogen-only hormone replacement therapy for a patient with an intact uterus
8   Prescribing methotrexate daily rather than weekly (unless initiated by a specialist for a specific clinical condition, for example, leukaemia)
9   A needle-stick injury caused by a failure to dispose of 'sharps' in compliance with national guidance and regulations
10 Adrenaline (or equivalent) is NOT available when clinically indicated for a medical emergency in the practice or GP home visit

---

There are problems with current incident reporting systems, the main ones being under-reporting or poorly specified reporting leading to selective and incomplete data, insufficient organisational expertise, investment and capacity to analyse the large number of reports generated, and finally a lack of focus on converting such analysis into improvement (WHO, 2020). Barriers to reporting include the confusion about what to report or who should report, individuals' sense of failure or fear of blame and litigation, reports being used out of context and lack of clarity about the benefits (NPSA, 2004b).

Reporting systems need a clear route to action from when an incident is reported and assessed to investigating causes, gaining insights into the system, and making recommendations for action to prevent future harm (WHO, 2020). As a result, the WHO developed the Minimal Information Model for Patient Safety Incident Reporting and Learning Systems (MIM PS), which involves two sections, structured and free text. The structured section includes patient information (age, sex), incident information (date, time, location, type, outcome), agents involved, suspected causes, contributing and mitigating factors, the reporter's role and resulting action. The idea of this is to focus on collectiing enough data to inform an investigation and analysis to inform learning and improvement.

INTEGRATED RISK MANAGEMENT AND PREVENTING SYSTEM FAILURE

Risk controls can reduce the chance of similar patient safety incidents occurring or reduce the potential for harm associated with a recurrence. Such controls include interventions at the level of the patient, healthcare staff, organisation, or health technologies for early detection, and the introduction of mitigating or ameliorating actions to reduce risk. Integrated risk management is a systematic approach to identifying, assessing, learning from and managing risk at an organisational level (NPSA, 2004b). This is achieved by combining risk management functions such as patient safety, patient complaints, litigation and health and safety, and aligning an organisation's clinical governance arrangements, business strategies, policies and activities to improve patient safety and outcomes.

The concept entails organisations having structures such as a board level risk management committee, local risk management groups, executive level and organisational experts and champions who are accountable for a coordinated approach to risk using risk assessment tools, probabilistic risk assessment, risk matrices and checklists. Failure Modes and Effects Analysis (FMEA) is a risk assessment tool that has been widely and successfully used (Liu et al., 2020) to identify processes (what is happening?), failure modes (what could go wrong?), contributory factors (why would it go wrong?) and effects (what are the consequences?).

BOX 5.2   STEPS OF A FAILURE MODES AND EFFECTS ANALYSIS (FMEA)

Identify a high-risk process
Form a team to analyse the process
Describe how the process can fail
Identify consequences and effects of the failure
Develop a risk matrix for each failure and its effects
Add risk controls to mitigate effects of failure
Construct and complete an action plan to implement the risk controls

---

PATIENT SAFETY MEASUREMENT TOOLS AND MEASURES

Most aspects of patient safety can and have been measured. Measurement methods include surveys of healthcare staff or patients, retrospective record reviews, some of which include trigger tools, checklists, voluntary reporting systems, active monitoring systems involving automated reviews of electronic records or administrative data, or simulated patients (Lydon et al., 2021) reviewing areas such as medications procedures and other treatments, laboratory testing and monitoring, care coordination, sentinel events, and facilities or resources (Hatoun et al., 2017).

Global trigger tools are instruments that are designed to identify, through record reviews, adverse events that result in 'additional monitoring, treatment, hospitalization, or death'. The reviews are done in two stages, the first a rapid screen, followed by a more detailed review (Hibbert et al., 2016). The commonest adverse events in a range of studies include infections, surgery or medication-related incidents, and the wide variation in rates (between 7% and 40% in inpatient settings) is often due to differences in how the tool is used (Hibbert et al., 2016).

The problems with current measures and measurements include variability of application and reporting, and the retrospective nature of many measures, detecting errors after an incident rather than preventing them (National Patient Safety Foundation, 2010).

━━━━━━━━━ **LEARNING ACTIVITY** ━━━━━━━━━

Measures and methods

Think about measuring patient safety, what you would measure and how you would go about this? How would you describe safety prevention in your organisation? What is the approach and how can you contribute to safer care?

SAFETY STRATEGIES, CULTURE AND CLIMATE

The Health Foundation's 'culture–behaviour–outcomes' model is a way of conceptualising the interrelationships between a range of different safety concepts including safety culture, climate, safety and outcomes (Health Foundation, 2011). Safety culture describes organisational values and actions related to patient safety; safety climate focuses on professional perceptions of the way in which safety is managed in an organisation; initiatives are changes implemented leading to improvements in health professional and patient outcomes. Previous studies have shown that the relationships between these are complex, often lacking or mixed, sometimes positive, and often bidirectional (DiCuccio, 2015; Hessels and Larson, 2016; Morello et al., 2013). Part of the problem lies in the fact that concepts such as safety culture (Waterson et al., 2019) and climate (Alsalem et al., 2018; Curran et al., 2018; Madden et al., 2022) are difficult to measure.

SAFETY TOOLS AND INTERVENTIONS: SAFETY CHECKLISTS, BRIEFINGS, HUDDLES, WALKROUNDS, HANDOVERS AND COLLABORATIVES

There have been several tools, methods or interventions used to improve patient safety. Arguably the best known of these is the checklist, which has been widely used in the aviation and other industries before being taken up in healthcare (Gawande, 2010). Most of these interventions, including the checklist, are complex interventions because they have multiple interacting components. They involve education to understand how and why the interventions should be applied as well as the intervention itself, which usually involves more than one person applying it.

The positive effects of checklists such as reduced incidence of adverse events and decreased mortality and morbidity are often mediated through improved compliance with guidelines, enhanced human factors such as teamwork and communication, together with other mechanisms that involve behaviour change that are only indirectly the result of the intervention itself (Boyd et al., 2017; McDowell and McComb, 2014; Russ et al., 2013; Thomassen et al., 2014).

Huddles are team discussions, often conducted daily to specifically identify and respond to safety risks, and have been found to be beneficial (Franklin et al., 2020). A development of this is the walkround, involving senior leadership visiting different areas of a hospital and meeting with staff to ask specific questions about adverse events or near misses, the factors that led to these events, and how future events are being mitigated (Frankel et al., 2003). There is some evidence that these are associated with better patient safety (Schwendimann et al., 2013) but also concerns that sometimes these are not always conducted in the way that they were intended because of attitudes of senior staff (Rotteau et al., 2014).

Communication is a vital aspect of these interventions, a particular example being handover of patients from one service or team to another, where structured handovers have been shown to improve communication and reduce the risk of miscommunication and errors (Bukoh and Siah, 2020; Muller et al., 2018).

Patient safety initiatives can also be scaled up and spread using techniques such as Quality Improvement Collaboratives whereby an expert group uses structured activities to engage healthcare teams to effect improvement in specific areas of practice. An example is shown in the case study in Box 5.3, 'Scaling up PINCER'.

BOX 5.3   CASE STUDY: SCALING UP PINCER (RODGERS ET AL., 2018)

Medication errors in general practice account for 5% of prescription items, with one in 550 items containing a potentially life-threatening error. They are important, expensive and a preventable cause of patient safety incidents causing illness, hospitalisations, and death.

A pharmacist-led information technology intervention for medication errors in general practice ('PINCER'), designed to search GP clinical systems using automated computerised prescribing safety indicators, identify patients at risk of prescription errors and correct these with pharmacist support, was found to be effective in a clinical trial and was therefore implemented in East Midlands UK general practices. Large-scale implementation involved a quality improvement collaborative, where an expert team, using structured activities, engaged clinicians and pharmacy teams to improve practice systems to reduce and prevent prescribing errors using education, feedback and pharmacist support.

Over just 18 months, between September 2015 and April 2017, PINCER was implemented in 370 general practices, searching almost 3 million patient records and identifying over 22,000 instances of potentially hazardous prescribing. Improvements in practice systems led to a reduction of 25% in the proportion of patients exposed to hazardous prescribing and this was reduced to around 10% after taking account of the natural fall in prescribing errors over time before PINCER was introduced. Reductions in hazardous prescribing were most apparent in drugs that increased the risk of gastrointestinal bleeding.

Further reading

Department of Health (2000) *An Organisation with a Memory: Report of an Expert Group on Learning from Adverse Events in the NHS*. London: The Stationery Office.

Donaldson, L., Ricciardi, W., Sheridan, S. and Tartaglia, R. (2021) *Textbook of Patient Safety and Clinical Risk Management*. Cham, Switzerland: Springer.

Kohn, L. T., Corrigan, J. and Donaldson, M. S. (2000) *To Err Is Human: Building a Safer Health System*. Washington, DC: National Academy Press.

NPSA (National Patient Safety Agency) (2004) *Seven Steps to Patient Safety: The Full Reference Guide*. London: NPSA

WHO (World Health Organization) (2009) Conceptual Framework for the International Classification for Patient Safety. Geneva: WHO. WHO/IER/PSP/2010.2.

WHO (World Health Organization) (2017) *Patient Safety: Making Health Care Safer*. Geneva: WHO. Document number WHO/HIS/SDS/2017.11.

┌─ Useful web resources ─┐

Health Education England. Patient safety. www.hee.nhs.uk/our-work/patient-safety
NHS England. Patient safety. www.england.nhs.uk/patient-safety/
The King's Fund. Patient safety. www.kingsfund.org.uk/topics/patient-safety
WHO (World Health Organization). Patient safety. www.who.int/health-topics/patient-safety

REFERENCES

Alsalem, G., Bowie, P. and Morrison, J. (2018) Assessing safety climate in acute hospital settings: a systematic review of the adequacy of the psychometric properties of survey measurement tools. *BMC Health Services Research,* 18 (1): 353.

Assiri, G. A., Shebl, N. A., Mahmoud, M. A., Aloudah, N., Grant, E., Aljadhey, H. and Sheikh, A. (2018) What is the epidemiology of medication errors, error-related adverse events and risk factors for errors in adults managed in community care contexts? A systematic review of the international literature. *BMJ Open,* 8 (5): e019101.

Bowie, P., Pope, L. and Lough, M. (2008) A review of the current evidence base for significant event analysis. *Journal of Evaluation in Clinical Practice,* 14 (4): 520–36.

Boyd, J., Wu, G. and Stelfox, H. (2017) The impact of checklists on inpatient safety outcomes: a systematic review of randomized controlled trials. *Journal of Hospital Medicine,* 12 (8): 675–82.

Bukoh, M. X. and Siah, C. R. (2020) A systematic review on the structured handover interventions between nurses in improving patient safety outcomes. *Journal of Nursing Management,* 28 (3): 744–55.

Council of the European Union (2009) European Council Recommendation on patient safety, including the prevention and control of healthcare associated infections. *Official Journal of the Europan Union,* Volume 52, 03 July: 2009/C 151/01. Retrieved from https://eur-lex.europa.eu/legal-content/EN/TXT/?uri=CELEX:320 09H0703(01).

Curran, C., Lydon, S., Kelly, M., Murphy, A., Walsh, C. and O'Connor, P. (2018) A systematic review of primary care safety climate survey instruments: their origins, psychometric properties, quality, and usage. *Journal of Patient Safety,* 14 (2): e9–e18.

de Vries, E. N., Ramrattan, M. A., Smorenburg, S. M., Gouma, D. J. and Boermeester, M. A. (2008) The incidence and nature of in-hospital adverse events: a systematic review. *Quality and Safety in Health Care,* 17 (3): 216–23.

de Wet, C., O'Donnell, C. and Bowie, P. (2014) Developing a preliminary 'never event' list for general practice using consensus-building methods. *British Journal of General Practice,* 64 (620): e159–67.

Department of Health (2000) *An Organisation with a Memory: Report of an Expert Group on Learning from Adverse Events in the NHS.* London: The Stationery Office.

DiCuccio, M. H. (2015) The relationship between patient safety culture and patient outcomes: a systematic review. *Journal of Patient Safety*, 11 (3): 135–42.

Dul, J., Bruder, R., Buckle, P., Carayon, P., Falzon, P., Marras, W. S., Wilson, J. R. and van der Doelen, B. (2012) A strategy for human factors/ergonomics: developing the discipline and profession. *Ergonomics*, 55 (4): 377–95.

Etchells, E., Koo, M., Daneman, N., McDonald, A., Baker, M., Matlow, A., Krahn, M. and Mittmann, N. (2012) Comparative economic analyses of patient safety improvement strategies in acute care: a systematic review. *BMJ Quality and Safety*, 21 (6): 448–56.

Frankel, A., Gandhi, T. K. and Bates, D. W. (2003) Improving patient safety across a large integrated health care delivery system. *International Journal for Quality in Health Care*, 15, Suppl 1, i31–i40.

Franklin, B. J., Gandhi, T. K., Bates, D. W., Huancahuari, N., Morris, C. A., Pearson, M., Bass, M. B. and Goralnick, E. (2020) Impact of multidisciplinary team huddles on patient safety: a systematic review and proposed taxonomy. *BMJ Quality and Safety*, 29 (10): 1–2.

Gawande, A. (2010) *The Checklist Manifesto: How to Get Things Right*. New York: Metropolitan Books.

Gillam, S. and Siriwardena, A. N. (2013) Frameworks for improvement: clinical audit, the plan-do-study-act cycle and significant event audit. *Quality in Primary Care*, 21 (2): 123–30.

Hagley, G., Mills, P. D., Watts, B. V. and Wu, A. W. (2019) Review of alternatives to root cause analysis: developing a robust system for incident report analysis. *BMJ Open Quality*, 8 (3): e000646.

Hatoun, J., Chan, J. A., Yaksic, E., Greenan, M. A., Borzecki, A. M., Shwartz, M. and Rosen, A. K. (2017) A systematic review of patient safety measures in adult primary care. *American Journal of Medical Quality*, 32 (3): 237–45.

Health Foundation (2011) *Does Improving Safety Culture Affect Patient Outcomes?* London: The Health Foundation. Retrieved from www.health.org.uk/publications/does-improving-safety-culture-affect-patient-outcomes.

Hegarty, J., Flaherty, S. J., Saab, M. M., Goodwin, J., Walshe, N., Wills, T., … Naughton, C. (2021) An international perspective on definitions and terminology used to describe serious reportable patient safety incidents: a systematic review. *Journal of Patient Safety*, 17 (8): e1247–54.

Hessels, A. J. and Larson, E. L. (2016) Relationship between patient safety climate and standard precaution adherence: a systematic review of the literature. *Journal of Hospital Infection*, 92 (4): 349–62.

Hibbert, P. D., Molloy, C. J., Hooper, T. D., Wiles, L. K., Runciman, W. B., Lachman, P., Muething, S. E. and Braithwaite, J. (2016) The application of the Global Trigger Tool: a systematic review. *International Journal of Quality in Health Care*, 28(6): 640–49.

Illich, I. (1977) *Limits to Medicine. Medical Nemesis: The Expropriation of Health* (new ed.). Harmondsworth and New York: Penguin.

Kellogg, K. M., Hettinger, Z., Shah, M., Wears, R. L., Sellers, C. R., Squires, M. and Fairbanks, R. J. (2017) Our current approach to root cause analysis: is it contributing to our failure to improve patient safety? *BMJ Quality and Safety*, 26 (5): 381–7.

Kohn, L. T., Corrigan, J. and Donaldson, M. S. (2000) *To Err Is Human: Building a Safer Health System*. Washington, DC: National Academy Press.

Laatikainen, O., Miettunen, J., Sneck, S., Lehtiniemi, H., Tenhunen, O. and Turpeinen, M. (2017) The prevalence of medication-related adverse events in inpatients – a systematic review and meta-analysis. *European Journal of Clinical Pharmacology*, 73 (12): 1539–49.

Lewis, P. J., Dornan, T., Taylor, D., Tully, M. P., Wass, V. and Ashcroft, D. M. (2009) Prevalence, incidence and nature of prescribing errors in hospital inpatients: a systematic review. *Drug Safety*, 32 (5): 379–89.

Liu, H. C., Zhang, L. J., Ping, Y. J. and Wang, L. (2020) Failure mode and effects analysis for proactive healthcare risk evaluation: a systematic literature review. *Journal of Evaluation in Clinical Practice*, 26 (4): 1320–37.

Lydon, S., Cupples, M. E., Murphy, A. W., Hart, N. and O'Connor, P. (2021) A systematic review of measurement tools for the proactive assessment of patient safety in general practice. *Journal of Patient Safety*, 2021, 17 (5): e406–e412.

Madden, C., Lydon, S., O'Dowd, E., Murphy, A. W. and O'Connor, P. (2022) A systematic review of patient-report safety climate measures in health care. *Journal of Patient Safety*, 18 (1): e51–e60.

Martin-Delgado, J., Martinez-Garcia, A., Aranaz-Andres, J. M., Valencia-Martin, J. L. and Mira, J. J. (2020) How much of Root Cause Analysis translates to improve patient safety. A systematic review. *Medical Principles and Practice*, 29 (6): 524–31.

McDowell, D. S. and McComb, S. A. (2014) Safety checklist briefings: a systematic review of the literature. *AORN Journal*, 99 (1), 125–37.

Mittmann, N., Koo, M., Daneman, N., McDonald, A., Baker, M., Matlow, A., Krahn, M., Shojania K. G. and Etchells, E. (2012) The economic burden of patient safety targets in acute care: a systematic review. *Drug Healthcare and Patient Safety*, 4: 141–65.

Morello, R. T., Lowthian, J. A., Barker, A. L., McGinnes, R., Dunt, D. and Brand, C. (2013) Strategies for improving patient safety culture in hospitals: a systematic review. *BMJ Quality and Safety*, 22 (1): 11–18.

Muller, M., Jurgens, J., Redaelli, M., Klingberg, K., Hautz, W. E. and Stock, S. (2018) Impact of the communication and patient hand-off tool SBAR on patient safety: a systematic review. *BMJ Open,* 8 (8), e022202.

National Patient Safety Foundation (2010) *Free from Harm: Accelerating Patient Safety Improvement Fifteen Years After To Err Is Human*. Boston, MA: National Patient Safety Foundation. Retrieved from www.ihi.org/resources/Pages/Publications/Free-from-Harm-Accelerating-Patient-Safety-Improvement.aspx

NPSA (National Patient Safety Agency) (2004a) National Reporting and Learning System (NRLS). Retrieved from https://report.nrls.nhs.uk/nrlsreporting/.

NPSA (National Patient Safety Agency) (2004b) *Seven Steps to Patient Safety: The Full Reference Guide*. London: NPSA

Omar, I., Graham, Y., Singhal, R., Wilson, M., Madhok, B. and Mahawar, K. K. (2021) Identification of common themes from never events data published by NHS England. *World Journal of Surgery*, 45 (3): 697–704.

Peerally, M. F., Carr, S., Waring, J. and Dixon-Woods, M. (2017) The problem with root cause analysis. *BMJ Quality and Safety*, 26 (5): 417–22.

Pringle, M. (2000) Significant event auditing. *Scandinavian Journal of Primary Health Care*, 18 (4): 200–2.

Reason, J. (1995). Understanding adverse events: human factors. *Quality in Health Care*, 4 (2): 80–9.

Reason, J. (2000) Human error: models and management. *BMJ*, 320 (7237): 768–70.

Reason, J. T., Carthey, J. and de Leval, M. R. (2001) Diagnosing 'vulnerable system syndrome': an essential prerequisite to effective risk management. *Quality in Health Care*, 10 Suppl 2: ii21–25.

Rodgers, S., Salema, N., Waring, J., Armstrong, S., Mehta, R., Bell, B., … Avery, A. (2018). *Improving Medication Safety in General Practices in the East Midlands through the PINCER Intervention: Scaling Up PINCER.* Evaluation Report for the Health Foundation. Retrieved from https://nottingham-repository.worktribe.com/output/1778784.

Rotteau, L., Shojania, K. G. and Webster, F. (2014) 'I think we should just listen and get out': a qualitative exploration of views and experiences of Patient Safety Walkrounds. *BMJ Quality and Safety*, 23 (10): 823–9.

Runciman, W. B., Williamson, J. A., Deakin, A., Benveniste, K. A., Bannon, K. and Hibbert, P. D. (2006) An integrated framework for safety, quality and risk management: an information and incident management system based on a universal patient safety classification. *Quality and Safety in Health Care*, 15 Suppl 1: i82–i90.

Russ, S., Rout, S., Sevdalis, N., Moorthy, K., Darzi, A. and Vincent, C. (2013) Do safety checklists improve teamwork and communication in the operating room? A systematic review. *Annals of Surgery*, 258 (6): 856–71.

Sari, A. A., Doshmangir, L. and Sheldon, T. (2010) A systematic review of the extent, nature and likely causes of preventable adverse events arising from hospital care. *Iranian Journal of Public Health*, 39 (3): 1–15.

Sattar, R., Johnson, J. and Lawton, R. (2020) The views and experiences of patients and health-care professionals on the disclosure of adverse events: a systematic review and qualitative meta-ethnographic synthesis. *Health Expectations*, 23 (3): 571–83.

Schwendimann, R., Milne, J., Frush, K., Ausserhofer, D., Frankel, A. and Sexton, J. B. (2013) A closer look at associations between hospital leadership walkrounds and patient safety climate and risk reduction: a cross-sectional study. *American Journal of Medical Quality*, 28 (5): 414–21.

Stocks, S. J., Alam, R., Bowie, P., Campbell, S., de Wet, C., Esmail, A. and Cheraghi-Sohi, S. (2019) Never events in UK general practice: a survey of the views of general practitioners on their frequency and acceptability as a safety improvement approach. *Journal of Patient Safety*, 15 (4): 334–42.

Sutherland, A., Canobbio, M., Clarke, J., Randall, M., Skelland, T. and Weston, E. (2020) Incidence and prevalence of intravenous medication errors in the UK: a systematic review. *European Journal of Hospital Pharmacy*, 27 (1), 3–8.

Thomassen, O., Storesund, A., Softeland, E.and Brattebo, G. (2014) The effects of safety checklists in medicine: a systematic review. *Acta Anaesthesiologica Scandinavica*, 58 (1): 5–18.

Vincent, C. A. (2004) Analysis of clinical incidents: a window on the system not a search for root causes. *Quality and Safety in Health Care*, 13 (4): 242–3.

Waterson, P., Carman, E. M., Manser, T. and Hammer, A. (2019) Hospital Survey on Patient Safety Culture (HSPSC): a systematic review of the psychometric properties of 62 international studies. *BMJ Open*, 9 (9): e026896.

WHO (World Health Organization) (2009) Conceptual Framework for the International Classification of Patient Safety. Geneva: WHO. WHO/IER/PSP/2010.2.

WHO (World Health Organization) (2017) *Patient Safety: Making Health Care Safer.* Geneva: WHO. Document number WHO/HIS/SDS/2017.11.

WHO (World Health Organization) (2019) Patient safety. Fact sheet. Retrieved from www.who.int/news-room/fact-sheets/detail/patient-safety.

WHO (World Health Organization) (2020) *Patient Safety Incident Reporting and Learning Systems: Technical Report and Guidance.* Geneva: WHO.

Williams, P. M. (2001). Techniques for root cause analysis. *Proceedings (Baylor University Medical Centre)*, 14 (2): 154–7.

6

PERSPECTIVES IN QUALITY IMPROVEMENT

Chapter summary

The aim of this chapter is to convey the range of perspectives that can underpin the theory, approach and practice of quality improvement. When there is an understanding of the perspectives and assumptions on our actions are based, we can also challenge these to give us scope for further improvement of what we do. Therefore, this chapter encourages the reader to think about their own ways of looking at the world and how this may influence their relationship with quality improvement.

Summary and learning points

- Why are perspectives important?
- What is a theory and how is it connected to perspectives?
- What are ontology and epistemology?
- What is a theory of change?
- Perspectives: business and management, psychological, sociological
- Theory versus practice and the importance of the interprofessional

WHY ARE PERSPECTIVES IMPORTANT?

A perspective is a way of looking at the world. The knowledge base and context which drive our point of view give us a sense of perspective. If we understand the factors that affect our standpoint, we can begin to unpick it, explore it and potentially challenge it. Typically, our standpoint can influence our decisions, how we behave and how we relate to others (Ayal et al., 2015). In quality improvement (QI), there is a range of perspectives and assumptions about what constitutes good quality of care and how to achieve it. In the spirit of quality improvement, by learning about our assumptions, and those of key stakeholders, we can reflect on our ways of thinking about and doing things, in order to continuously better them. It may also be that QI initiatives are taking place in a context with multiple stakeholders coming at a problem from different perspectives and, again, with differing agendas. By seeking to understand these perspectives, we can gauge the extent to which our QI initiative can meet the needs of its stakeholders and where compromises need to be reached. Before outlining a number of perspectives, the next part of this chapter will clarify a number of key concepts related to the idea of perspectives.

WHAT IS A THEORY AND HOW IS IT CONNECTED TO PERSPECTIVES?

A theory is a collection of ideas that have the aim of explaining a particular phenomenon. Typically, a theory is a set of general principles that can be used to explain why and how certain things occur (Asher, 1984). When it comes to academia, theories are created to substantiate, as well as challenge, the ways in which we look at the world. By using theories to scaffold research findings, we can contribute to knowledge. Therefore, a theory can help inform and shape our perspectives. Theories can also become popularised and enter into popular culture and parlance. For instance, elements of psychoanalytical Freudian theory, such as 'repression', 'hysteria' and 'ego' have entered the realm of how features of our emotional life may be conceptualised. We therefore end up being influenced by theoretical constructs without conscious awareness of it (another Freudian theoretical concept!). Within the realm of quality improvement, it is therefore important to understand whether certain theoretical assumptions about what constitutes quality and ways of looking at the world are driving our ways of doing things. Further, it may be worth revisiting theoretical constructs to help us understand how quality improvement is (or isn't) being enacted, including the contributory factors to its success (or lack thereof).

WHAT ARE ONTOLOGY AND EPISTEMOLOGY?

Ontology and epistemology are constructs related to perspectives, theory and theoretical perspectives. They may be relatively complex to understand and unlikely to be considered in day-to-day quality improvement implementation. However, they tend to be important in scholarly enquiry and for those readers who may wish to teach or conduct research in the future, or already do. **Ontology** is a branch of philosophy concerned with the enquiry into being, the human existence and how reality is conceived. Ontology is also the study of how phenomena are classified, what they do and do not have in common and how they relate to one another. Guba and Lincoln (1994) propose that ontological enquiry seeks to understand the nature of reality and the knowledge that can be gained about reality. In relation to quality improvement, we can consider the opposing influences of objectivism and subjectivism. Through the ontological lens of objectivism, there is an assumption that quality exists in a factual, objective form, independent of the agendas of others, and understood to be ever-present, as a measurable construct. On the other hand, subjectivism implies that reality is the product of human experiences and perceptions. Therefore, it can be argued that what we conceive to be 'quality' in health is socially constructed (Harteloh, 2003). Typically, QI initiatives have taken an objectivist standpoint – namely, that quality is a measurable, objectively observed entity. It may be that this ontological perspective precludes quality improvement experts from building an appreciation of the more messy reality of quality and quality improvement – namely less predictable people and contextual factors, such as staff levels of acceptance of the QI initiative and sociopolitical influences such as government policy and funding allocation for instance. Therefore, it may be that an awareness of a range of ontological perspectives helps to shape quality improvement implementation that is more suitable for and adaptive to the 'real' world.

Epistemology is another branch of philosophy concerned with the theory of knowledge. In other words, what is the origin and nature of what we know and how do we justify it? How is it that we acquire knowledge? In relation to quality improvement, we may be interested in how we know what we know about quality and its improvement and if there are ways for us to challenge this and enhance it further for more effective quality improvement implementation. In seeking an epistemological understanding, we may wish to know what our assumptions and justifications are for the ways in which we design quality improvement. For instance, if we believe clinicians to hold key expertise in care delivery, this may preclude us from involving patients to co-produce QI programmes, missing out on the expert knowledge of those with lived experience. Though by no means exhaustive, the next part of the chapter will outline several perspectives that are likely to underpin quality improvement, either in isolation, but more typically as a combination of different beliefs and world views as to what constitutes quality and the enactment of quality improvement.

WHAT IS A THEORY OF CHANGE?

A 'theory of change' is a detailed description of the assumptions about why and how a desired change will happen. In healthcare quality improvement, health quality improvers assume that a particular QI intervention, such as team training for instance, will lead to improved patient experience. Therefore, improvers hold a theory at the core of their work, which is that what one ends up with will be better than what one started with prior to quality improvement taking place. However, by building a theory of change through drawing on a range of stakeholder viewpoints, we can begin to challenge our underpinning assumptions and evaluate the success of our change. It may be that the patients who contribute their views to the theory of change are unanimous in how knowledgeable their clinicians are, but it is the quality of waiting areas which affects their level of satisfaction. Therefore, a theory of change could lead improvers to prioritising the use of resources towards an overhaul of the waiting areas over team training in order to create more likelihood of an improvement in patient satisfaction. A theory of change can be illustrated through gathering information in relation to the following areas of interest: input (such as cost and time), output (such as health information sessions), outcomes (such as change in patient health indicators), impact (such as improved population health) and social value (such as reduction in health inequalities).

PERSPECTIVES

Business and management

Business and management thinking features highly in the field of quality improvement, in particular the manufacturing roots of operationalisable QI approaches such as Lean. Business and management as a discipline is concerned with the study of the coordination and organisation of business activities, as well as with contributing to theoretical approaches around management, including related areas such as leadership, followership (i.e. the study of those being led) and human resource management. Further, taking a business and management view of quality improvement could be underpinned by a series of business principles. There is a range of viewpoints and ways of defining what principles a business should be driven by. For instance, the Financial Conduct Authority (the main regulator of financial markets in the UK), lists management and control, and financial prudence as two of its 11 business principles. In which case, quality improvement may be viewed through the lens of business and management as a defined linear process that requires close oversight and control, ensuring that resources are utilised in the most efficient way. This has parallels with health economic perspectives of quality improvement, which are concerned with the allocation of resources. In the context of a publicly owned healthcare service as in the UK, this relates to best use of taxation, including investment in the development of new treatments, as well as the equity of access nationally for all citizens. Health economists may ask the question of what QI initiative achieves best value for money for the taxpayer and provides a return on investment. In the case of healthcare, will a particular initiative reduce costs in the long run, for instance by better workforce planning or through improving patient outcomes in the long term?

Here merely an overview of a handful of perspectives that could underpin quality improvement is presented. One recent development within quality improvement, stemming from an area of business and management, is the application of socio-technical systems to quality improvement. Socio-technical systems refer to the marrying up of the social aspects of an organisation, alongside the technical elements, such as its structure and processes. Therefore, in basic terms, socio-technical systems as a theoretical approach is concerned with the interaction between people and the technical. In quality improvement, given the complexity of healthcare, the physical design of tools and technologies is important, but Carayon (2012) notes that if the understanding of the organisational context within which these tools are used is lacking, then staff 'may develop work-arounds and the tools may not be used safely', in turn affecting patient safety. Carayon argues for the socio-technical systems approach, therefore, to give rise to targeted QI initiatives, based on an awareness of the broader system within which they are implemented.

There is an overlap here with human factors, which straddle business and management and psychological perspectives. Human factors as a discipline is concerned with three interrelated areas of people in industry – the job, the individual and the organisation. The key premise of human factors is that change programmes will not be effective if only one of these areas in considered in isolation. Therefore, through the lens of human factors, in quality improvement, it is crucial to know what task people are being asked to do, who is doing it and whether they have the knowledge and capability to carry out the task effectively, and where they are working, both the organisation and the societal context within which the organisation operates.

The extent to which business and management perspectives, particularly those more closely aligned to manufacturing, are applicable to healthcare quality improvement has been questioned. In the instance of Lean (a production method focused on eliminating waste in the system, which is described in more detail in Chapter 7), there may be a range of organisational barriers and enablers to its successful implementation. A literature review from 2010 (Mazzocato et al., 2010) draws on the research evidence to argue that Lean in healthcare is typically applied to small-scale technical scenarios, rather than large-scale organisational transformation. In a study of a transformational programme in imaging (Radcliffe et al., 2020), we found that imaging, given its more routinised and standardised care processes, was fertile ground for lean implementation, with high levels of 'buy in' from radiology staff. In line with socio-technical systems theory, we argued that attention needs to be paid to the context of Lean implementation, as well as interprofessional relationships. Yet, Radnor and colleagues (2012) highlight the utility of Lean on a micro rather than a macro level, along with the poor fit of a manufacturing management solution to the healthcare context overall. Nonetheless, barriers to Lean implementation may not always be specific to the healthcare context. Jørgensen and Emmitt (2008) highlight the issues of applying Lean to the construction industry and the difficulties outlined are not dissimilar to those cited in the healthcare literature. It may be that taking manufacturing-specific or business and management approaches more broadly to other settings without adaptation can bring about some contextual misalignment.

Psychological

Psychology is the study of behaviour and the mind. As a discipline, its interest is focused on how people think, feel, act and interact. Therefore, in the context of quality improvement, a psychological perspective would be centred on the individual and group human activities leading to improvement or otherwise, and how interpersonal facets of teams and organisations may impact on the implementation of QI. Further, Bonin (2018) argues that psychologists need to have a greater presence in healthcare quality improvement, both through applying QI principles to their own work, as well as in playing a role in organisational development and systems redesign. In contrast to classical industrial approaches to quality improvement, Godfrey and colleagues (2014) claim that improvement in health is 80% human and only 20% technical. Thus, factors including staff disengagement and lack of support are likely to impinge on the success of an improvement intervention.

A psychological theoretical perspective of quality improvement would take into account the thoughts and feelings of those implementing the improvement and how their wellbeing could best be supported. It may be that team members actively or inadvertently seek to undermine the QI initiative, for instance, through gaming. Gaming may be a response to the standardisation in healthcare through quality improvement, namely manipulating outputs of performance metrics (Kordowicz and Ashworth, 2010). Gaming may reflect a level of disengagement with the QI frameworks and a desire to discredit their usefulness, whereby participants work to only the target threshold required and some even go so far as to distort the output, rather than use the framework as a legitimate means of improving their clinical performance. Psychological theory may help us to understand unintended phenomena such as gaming, for instance by drawing on motivation theory, including what incentivises us most effectively to perform at work, or psychological under-standings of employee engagement.

Further, it is of importance to psychologists interested in the organisation to identify how people work together, what their professional relationships are like, and the type of organisational culture within which they operate. Chapter 8 of this book explores the subject of relational quality improvement in greater depth. Mannion and Davies (2018) argue that the culture of an organisation is a collec-tion of shared ways of thinking, feeling and behaviour and that this can impact on quality improvement efforts. However, they convey the complexity of health-care organisations, which often comprise multiple subcultures either increasing or undermining the impact of quality improvement. They therefore call for a more nuanced approach to understanding the cultural dynamics in the delivery of healthcare. Here, sociology is another perspective, which too can play an important role in how quality improvement is approached.

Sociological

Sociology is the study of society, social interactions between humans and human behaviour within societies, as well as of culture. Indeed, Everett Rogers (2003), who popularised the notion of diffusion of innovation (i.e. how innovative and new ways of working and technological innovations become adopted and spread – diffuse – over time), claimed that 'an innovation is communicated through certain channels over time among the members of a social system' (p. 5). Therefore, its application to quality improvement would be a concern with how social systems impact on quality and how they can be the drivers of or constraining factors in improvement. In addition, it has been argued that simply the focus on enablers and barriers is reductionist in its oversimplifications of social science research. Zuiderent-Jerak and colleagues (2009) posit that instead the multiple ontologies that social sciences can bring to understanding quality improvement, such as through getting under the skin of policy agendas and what constitutes the imple-mentation of effective care and the consequence of these multifaceted approaches for patient safety, are the key advantage of applying a sociological lens to quality improvement. A seminal paper by DiMaggio and Powell (1983) coined the soci-ological term 'institutional isomorphism'. They argued that there are a range of mechanisms or institutional pressures that cause organisations within a particular field to become homogenous, or isomorphic. It could be that standardised qual-ity improvement approaches lead to homogenous healthcare organisations. Whilst arguments in support of this may suggest that this leads to equitable healthcare, the sociological theory of institutional isomorphism proposes that this is a constrain-ing phenomenon, where if organisational units resemble one another, this may not take into account contextual factors, whilst stifling innovation and creativity, and ignoring difference in cultural traditions and local need. Therefore, institutional isomorphism suggests that tailored, individualised and person-centred approaches to quality improvement, are more likely to give rise to positive processes and action.

It is also of relevance to consider the medical sociology perspective. Medical sociology, a branch of sociology, is the study of the social factors, causes and conse-quences of health and illness, including the delivery of health. The interest in how the social environment affects human health grew in the post-war climate, where unsurprisingly much deliberation socio-politically was given to the best allocation of scarce resources. Medical sociology helped to highlight how social processes and institutions impact on public health, as well as patient and professional perspec-tives of health and illness. Whilst Allen and others (2015) argue that sociology has a key role to play in improving healthcare quality, they recognise that what can be perceived as a somewhat detached critical and complex stance of sociologists may seem too removed from practice and lacking in the quick fix preferred by managers. Sociological understandings may also challenge widely accepted 'tropes' in qual-ity improvement, moving towards more effective conceptualisations of how qual-ity improvement is enacted. For instance, Zuiderent-Jerak (2009) and colleagues unpick concepts such as 'effectiveness' and 'client participation' and argue for their reframing through sociological study in order to move towards solving QI issues. Lastly, key theorists have advocated for a 'sociology of quality improvement and patient safety', in other words, a sociological theory of quality improvement and patient safety as a freestanding field of enquiry (Allen et al., 2016). It is through the sociology of quality improvement that complex social dilemmas can be unpicked in order to progress not only the theory, but also the practice, of quality and safety in healthcare.

THEORY VERSUS PRACTICE AND THE IMPORTANCE OF THE INTERPROFESSIONAL

It is more than likely that quality improvement will take place in a 'messy' context – one where multiple systemic factors and stakeholders' perspectives have to be taken into consideration, whilst leaving space for unpredictable events and contingencies. Therefore, this raises the question as to the extent to which one theory can provide a sound underpinning framework for effective QI efforts. It may be the case that integrated approaches, drawing on a range of disciplines in health and social care, are more likely to breed real-world impact. In particular, the current policy context is seeing a move towards Integrated Care Systems – partnerships of health and social care organisations, working collaboratively to deliver joined up (rather than frag-mented) care around the patient in order to improve health outcomes and narrow health inequalities (Goodwin et al., 2012). Reducing strain on resources and pooling knowledge through different professions working together are the key drivers of multi- and interdisciplinary approaches to delivering healthcare. There is a body of literature indicating the advantages of interprofessional training and working to help improve the quality and safety of care. For instance, there is a link between effective interprofessional working and staff retention (Baik and Zierler, 2019), as well as in helping to tackle what Berwick and others (2008) describe as the triple aim – the experience of care, improved population health and reducing healthcare cost per capita.

Furthermore, we can pose the question of whether drawing on the experiential achieved through practice, rather than theoretical musings, is likely to be of greater importance when it comes to understanding and implementing quality improvement in the 'real world'. Indeed, whilst a theory is merely a proposed explanation of why something happens or may occur, practice refers to the actual doing. Therefore, it can be argued that practical knowledge can be more valuable than theoretical knowledge as it is gained through contextual and situated experience. Briner and colleagues (2009) argue that management practice needs to stem from an evidence-base, but that experience too is an important part of how that evidence base is built up over time. Importantly, socially situated knowledge also calls on us to be aware of the power dynamics at play within our context, such as how our social positioning and protected characteristics (e.g. age, race, beliefs, etc.) can shape and influence what we know and how we apply our knowledge.

Further reading

Koontz, H. (1961) The management theory jungle. *Journal of the Academy of Management*, 4 (3): 174–88.
Rogers, E (2003) *Diffusion of Innovations*, 5th ed. New York: Free Press.

REFERENCES

Allen, D., Braithwaite, J., Sandall, J. and Waring, J. (2016) Towards a sociology of healthcare safety and quality. *Sociology of Health and Illness*, 38 (2): 181–97.

Asher, H. B. (1984) *Theory-Building and Data Analysis in the Social Sciences*. Knoxville, TN: University of Tennessee Press.

Ayal, S., Rusou, Z., Zakay, D. and Hochman, G. (2015) Determinants of judgment and decision making quality: the interplay between information processing style and situational factors. *Frontiers in Psychology*, 6: 1088.

Baik, D. and Zierler, B. (2019) RN job satisfaction and retention after an interprofessional team intervention. *Western Journal of Nursing Research*, 41 (4): 615–30.

Berwick, D. M., Nolan, T. W. and Whittington, J. (2008) The triple aim: care, health, and cost. *Health Affairs (Project Hope)*, 27 (3): 759–69.

Bonin, L. (2018) Quality improvement in health care: the role of psychologists and psychology. *Journal of Clinical Psychology in Medical Settings*, 25 (3): 278–94.

Briner, R., Denyer, D. and Rousseau, D. (2009) Evidence-based management: concept cleanup time? *Academy of Management Perspectives*, 23: 19–32.

Carayon P. (2012) Sociotechnical systems approach to healthcare quality and patient safety. *Work (Reading, Mass.)*, 41, Suppl 1 (0 1): 3850–4.

DiMaggio, P. J. and Powell, W. W. (1983) The Iron Cage revisited: institutionalisomorphism and collective rationality in organizational fields. *American Sociological Review*, 48 (2): 147–60.

Godfrey, M., Andersson-Gare, B., Nelson, E. C., Nilsson, M. and Ahlstrom, G. (2014) Coaching interprofessional health care improvement teams: the coachee, the coach and the leader perspectives. *Journal of Nursing Management*, 22 (4): 452–64.

Goodwin, N., Smith, J., Davies, A., Perry, C., Rosen, R., Dixon, A., Dixon, J. and Ham, C. (2012) *Integrated Care for Patients and Populations: Improving Outcomes by Working Together: A Report to the Department of Health and the NHS Future Forum.* London: The King's Fund.

Guba, E. G. and Lincoln, Y. S. (1994) Competing paradigms in qualitative research. In N. K. Denzin and Y. S. Lincoln (eds), *Handbook of Qualitative Research.* Thousand Oaks, CA: Sage Publications, Inc. pp. 105–17.

Harteloh, P. (2003) The meaning of quality in health care: a conceptual analysis. *Health Care Analysis*, 11 (3): 259–67.

Jørgensen, B. and Emmitt, S. (2008) Lost in transition: the transfer of lean manufacturing to construction. *Engineering, Construction and Architectural Management*, 15 (4): 383–98.

Kordowicz, M. and Ashworth, M. (2010) Smoke and mirrors? Informatics opportunities and challenges of the Quality and Outcomes Framework. In N. Siriwardena and S. Gillam (eds), *How the Quality and Outcomes Framework Is Transforming General Practice.* Oxford: Radcliffe.

Mannion, R. and Davies, H. (2018) Understanding organisational culture for healthcare quality improvement. *BMJ*, 363; k4907.

Mazzocato, P., Savage, C., Brommels, M., Aronsson, H. and Thor, J. (2010) Lean thinking in healthcare: a realist review of the literature. *BMJ Quality and Safety*, 19: 376–82.

Radcliffe, E., Kordowicz, M., Mak, C., Shefer, G., Armstrong, D., White, P. and Ashworth, M. (2020) Lean implementation within healthcare: imaging as fertile ground. *Journal of Health Organization and Management*, Oct 14; ahead-of-print. doi: 10.1108/JHOM-02-2020-0050.

Radnor, Z., Holweg, M. and Waring, J. (2012) Lean in healthcare: The unfilled promise? *Social Science and Medicine*, 74 (3): 364–71.

Rogers, E. (2003) *Diffusion of Innovations*, 5th ed. New York: Free Press.

Zuiderent-Jerak, T., Starting, M., Nieboer, A. and Bal, R. (2009) Sociological refigurations of patient safety; ontologies of improvement and 'acting with' quality collaboratives in healthcare. *Social Science and Medicine*, 69 (12): 1713–21.

SECTION C

APPROACHES, MODELS AND TOOLKITS

7

TROUBLESHOOTING AND OPERATIONALISING QUALITY IMPROVEMENT

Chapter summary

Quality improvement is a troubleshooting activity involving identifying and understanding problems and solving them using knowledge of what works and how it works in different contexts using a range of tools that have been developed for the purpose.

This chapter defines what we mean by troubleshooting in the context of quality improvement, explains how to identify and analyse problems and presents methods for developing and implementing solutions.

It presents and critically analyses the main approaches and tools for quality improvement and the theories underpinning them, ranging from simpler to more complex interventions using multiple techniques to problem solving.

Summary and learning points

- Definitions
- Identifying problems
- Understanding and analysing processes

- The importance of theories, models and frameworks for planning improvement
- Developing solutions
- Methods for problem solving
- Clinical audit
- The model for improvement
- The 'Plan–Do–Study–Act' (PDSA) cycle
- Lean management
- Six Sigma

DEFINITIONS

Troubleshooting is the act of 'analysing and solving' problems (Oxford English Dictionary). On the surface, this might be taken to imply that we only need to undertake quality improvement when there is a problem. But that type of thinking is a problem in itself since anything can be improved. As Deming (2000) pointed out, 'If you can't describe what you are doing as a process, you don't know what you're doing.'

So, for the purpose of quality improvement as far as this chapter is concerned, troubleshooting is the act of 'analysing and improving' processes. In Chapter 3 we learned why we should improve healthcare quality while in this chapter we focus on how to improve it.

In order to improve healthcare quality, we first need to appreciate that healthcare is a process or set of processes. Processes, built on structures, lead to outputs and outcomes. To bring about improvements we need to understand these processes in depth. We also need to be clear what outputs and outcomes we are aiming for and how these can be operationalised and measured. Finally, we need to know how to change processes to bring about the intended improvements and to measure outputs and outcomes to see whether change has been brought about.

There are several different approaches to troubleshooting for quality improvement, including clinical audit, significant event analysis or techniques such as Lean, Six Sigma, and combinations of these such as Lean Six Sigma.

IDENTIFYING PROBLEMS

The first step in troubleshooting is to identify that there is a problem with healthcare delivery processes or outcomes. Difficulties with care can be revealed as poor measures of processes or outcomes of care. Measures or criteria of care can be evidence-based, sometimes termed review criteria, for example if processes are known to relate directly to outcomes or if outcomes are important to patients or both.

Problems can be identified in different ways, including through safety events and learning from these using root cause, critical incident or significant event analysis (see Chapter 5). Alternatively, performance might be seen as suboptimal through research, the baseline findings from an audit or quality improvement project, or a benchmarking exercise, which can show gaps in expected performance in relation to evidence of best practice, agreed standards or in comparison with others, respectively. Standards can be informed by published evidence, grey literature, or the highest or average performance achieved, whether by different professionals, teams or organisations.

━━━━━━━━━━━━━ **LEARNING ACTIVITY** ━━━━━━━━━━━━━

Problems in your healthcare practice

Think about a problem you have experienced in your practice. What was the problem? How was this identified? How did this affect the care provided? What was the evidence for best practice?

UNDERSTANDING AND ANALYSING PROCESSES

The next step to solving problems with health care is to analyse these problems in detail to understand how they have arisen and how they may be overcome. In terms of the Donabedian quality domains (Donabedian, 1966) this includes understanding the structures (people, plant, property), processes and outcomes (effectiveness, safety and experience) of care.

According to Deming, one of the founding fathers of quality improvement, 'Every activity, every job is part of a process' (Deming, 2000), and healthcare is no exception. The importance of process has been emphasised by others, including Balestracci, who in stating that 'all work is a process' points to breakdowns and inconsistencies in work processes in the context of the wider system as the source of failures in quality (Balestracci and Medical Group Management Association, 2015). Juran in his *Quality Handbook* devotes a chapter to process management, and the notion of Process Quality Management (PQM), in which the process is defined in relation to the needs of the service user, outcomes are measured in relation to the process and the process is redesigned to produce better outcomes (Juran and Godfrey, 1998).

The first step is to understand the current process. To achieve this, a set of techniques called process mapping has been developed for understanding healthcare or other processes in detail. Process mapping seeks to understand, with those involved, the detail of how healthcare is provided, including what happens, when and how, and who receives or does not receive care, as well as how it achieves its effects.

A systematic review of process mapping in healthcare has helped us to understand its key phases and features. The first phase involves identification of the process to be examined and the stakeholders, including professional and patient representatives, who will help to do this; the second phase involves gathering data and information to inform the process mapping; the third phase seeks to gather a range of perspectives to help generate a map using sticky notes; and the fourth final phase is where the map is analysed, further information gathered, the paper version is transferred to computer and the map is validated or agreed by stakeholders and other informants (Antonacci et al., 2021).

Reasons for examining a particular process can vary but could include concerns about failures, safety or cost, a need to reduce identified variation, or response to regulatory requirements. Those involved in delivering or receiving the process need to be involved in the process mapping exercise, because whether change happens, whether it is well designed to lead to improvement and whether potential improvements are relevant and important to those receiving it are all critical.

Describing the process will usually mean interacting in some way with stakeholders involved, to gather detailed information on the process, what is involved and how it operates. Steps in the process and how these occur, whether through thought processes, actions or interactions, are drawn in flow charts, called process maps. Sometimes cause-and-effect diagrams are used to show how various processes can underlie a particular problem or phenomenon.

BOX 7.1 TECHNIQUES FOR ANALYSING, DISPLAYING AND IMPROVING PROCESSES

Understanding and analysing processes

1 Individual interviews (discovery, narrative) or focus groups
2 Patient or practitioner self-administered surveys
3 Direct observation

Displaying processes

1 Process maps
2 Cause-and-effect ('fishbone') diagram

Improving the process

1 Critical-to-quality (CTQ) tree
2 Driver diagram

The Ambulance Services Cardiovascular Quality Initiative (ACSQI), a national quality improvement collaborative for improving prehospital ambulance care for heart attack (acute myocardial infarction) and stroke in England (Siriwardena et al., 2014), used a range of techniques from those listed (see Figure 7.1). These included patient interviews to understand barriers and facilitators to improvement. Quality improvement (QI) teams in each ambulance service supported by a national coordinating expert group organised workshops in each service to conduct process mapping which generated CTQ trees and cause-and-effect diagrams designed to understand how best to improve processes. Finally, Plan–Do–Study–Act cycles were undertaken to test these interventions in rapid cycle tests of change which were monitored using statistical process control (SPC) charts. Learning was shared

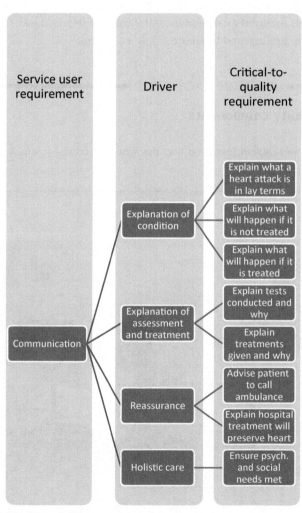

Figure 7.1 Critical-to-quality tree example

between QI teams who met together at three national workshops, between QI leads through monthly teleconferences, and between the expert group and participants.

The interviews of patients found that good communication (explanation of the condition, clinical assessments and treatment, reassurance and holistic care), effective and professional treatment (including good pain management and professionalism), and smooth transitions of care (timeliness of arrival and treatment, the journey to hospital and a good handover at hospital) were critical to quality (Togher et al., 2013). This could have been supplemented by patient surveys or direct observations of care.

A CTQ tree identifies three things: a service user requirement or need, the driver or drivers of this requirement broken down into action points and the critical-to-quality requirements to meet the driver. A CTQ tree was used to summarise patients' needs for good quality prehospital care for heart attack. The communication domain is summarised in Figure 7.1 as a CTQ tree.

━━━━━ LEARNING ACTIVITY ━━━━━

Critical quality components

Think about the problem identified and describe the critical-to-quality aspects of the process.

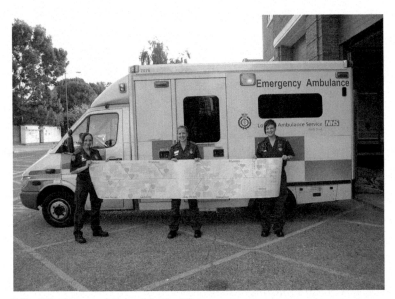

Figure 7.2   What a process map looks like

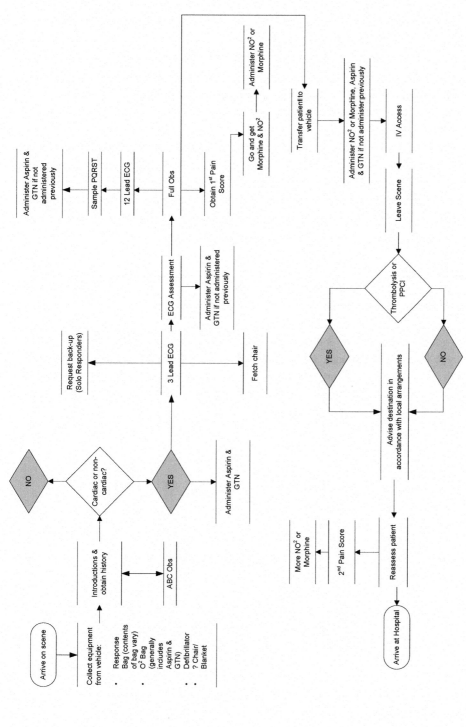

Figure 7.3 Process map showing prehospital care for heart attack

Process mapping involves front-line staff using visual methods including diagrams, flowcharts, or algorithms, to describe a process in detail in order to improve it. The process can be mapped on a board (nowadays most often a whiteboard) or large piece of paper, and commonly this uses sticky notes. For example, in the ASCQI project. process mapping was undertaken at workshops in each ambulance service to describe the processes in place and to determine how these might be improved.

Once a process map is developed using these traditional approaches, it can be transferred to a computerised image for further development, discussion and use (Figure 7.3).

Problems in a process, including explanations for defects or variation, can be summarised in a cause-and-effect (fishbone, Ishikawa) diagram (Figure 7.4) which incorporates the problem to be solved at the head of the fish to the right and the causes forming the skeleton to left (Figure 7.4). An example from the ASCQI project is shown in Figure 7.5. Finally, these can inform the means of improving care based on theory to develop solutions to the problems found.

━━━━━━ LEARNING ACTIVITY ━━━━━━

Analysing the process

Think about the problem identified. Describe the steps in the process that should have happened in detail. Consider the contributions of patients, healthcare providers, policies and equipment as well as process steps to the problem. What factors contributed to the problem and how could these have been prevented? How might the process be simplified while retaining critical-to-quality components?

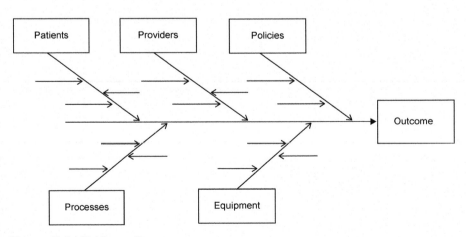

Figure 7.4　Fishbone diagram

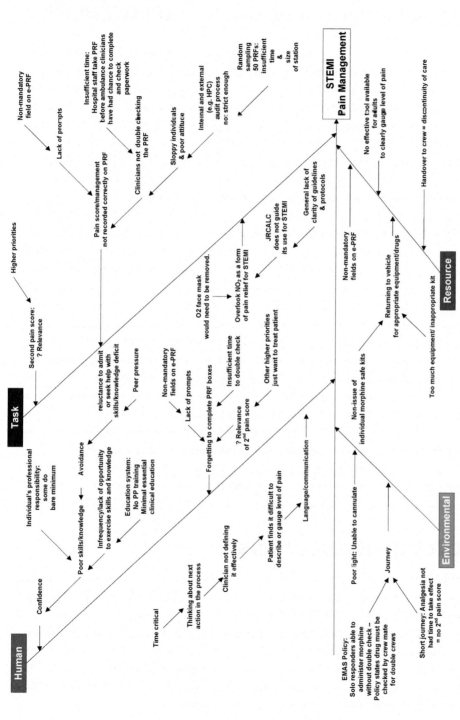

Figure 7.5 Fishbone diagram of pain management in heart attack

THE IMPORTANCE OF THEORIES, MODELS AND FRAMEWORKS FOR PLANNING IMPROVEMENT

As explored in Chapter 6, theory is often considered rather abstract when we are thinking about solutions to problems, but theory is critical to understanding how to improve care. A theory is 'a set of propositions that are logically related, expressing the relation(s) among several different constructs and propositions' (Varpio et al., 2020). It has also been defined as 'a set of analytical principles or statements designed to structure our observation, understanding and explanation of the world (Nilsen, 2015).

Theory, in the context of quality improvement, can mean anything from hunches (working hypotheses), to middle range theory which integrates empirical research with broader theory (e.g. normalisation process theory), to grand (e.g. social, psychological, behavioural) social and scientific theories. Each individually or in combination may help to inform the problem under consideration. Programme theories are considered to underpin logic models and include a combination of theories that help to explain how changes in activities, structures or processes might affect outcomes. These are usually based on previous evidence but could also be based on a hunch about what might work. The key is that they need to be formulated in a way which can be tested to show whether they work or do not, i.e. they are amenable to 'falsification' in the language of Popper and the scientific method (Popper, 2002).

An excellent way to understand theory from a quality improvement perspective is the 'coin spinning game (or exercise)' developed by Dr David Williams. The game involves teams of people competing to see how long they can spin a coin. Each team is given a selection of coins of different sizes and weights with a description of the aim of the game. Teams are tasked with using their experience or hunches as a group to generate ideas for how they can keep a coin spinning for the longest period of time. Once these potential solutions are generated, they test these hypotheses (e.g. modifying size or weight or coin or surface, etc.) by trying out each option in turn, measuring the time that the coin spins and recording this on a chart, such as a run chart.

DEVELOPING SOLUTIONS

Possible ways to improve processes can be developed from theory or working hypotheses. Theories for improvement might include theories of learning (e.g. behaviourist, cognitive, humanistic, transformative, social, motivational, reflective) (Taylor and Hamdy, 2013), behaviour change (Francis et al., 2012), implementation (e.g. diffusion of innovation theory; Rogers, 2003), normalisation process theory (Murray et al., 2010) or a wide range of other theories and theoretical frameworks for implementation or improvement, for example the Consolidated Framework for Implementation Research (Damschroder et al., 2009).

In the ASCQI study (Siriwardena et al., 2014), cited previously, various learning and behavioural theories or hypotheses were used as a basis for actions and interventions, some of which, including educational outreach, audit, feedback and reminders, were supported by published evidence (Johnson and May, 2015). Other approaches, for example realist methods (Pawson, 2013), can also be used to develop working hypotheses for improvement (Cooper et al., 2019).

The shared ideas for testing developed by a team or organisation can be summarised in a driver diagram. In the diagram the aim is specified and is supported by a number of primary drivers, each arising from one or more secondary drivers, built on change ideas and change concepts (Bennett and Provost, 2015). An example from the ASCQI project is shown in Figure 7.6.

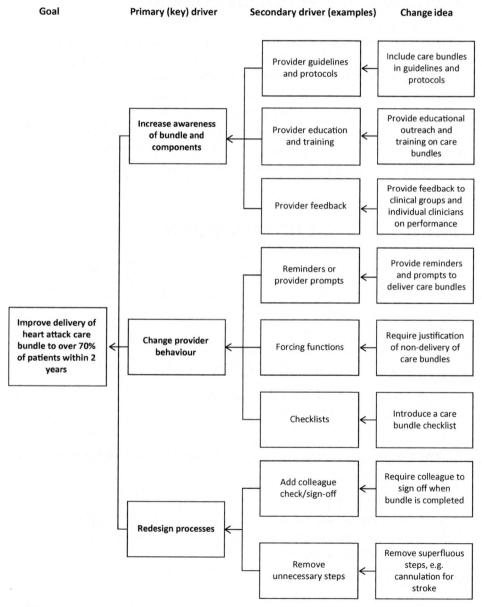

Figure 7.6   Driver diagram to improve reliability of prehospital care for heart attack

━━━━━━━━━━━ LEARNING ACTIVITY ━━━━━━━━━━━

Problem solving

Think about the problem identified. Use a theory, framework or model to generate possible solutions.

METHODS FOR PROBLEM SOLVING

Over the past decades, a number of methods have been developed for solving problems. Although they each use different philosophical and theoretical approaches or vary in the activities they adopt, they are largely based on similar principles. These include leadership and teamwork in support of continuous quality improvement, which involves identifying the problem or problems to be solved, setting goals or aims, understanding and analysing the processes involved, using theory to develop possible solutions, using experiments to test these, measuring their effects, and making efforts to sustain improvement where it occurs.

THE MODEL FOR IMPROVEMENT

The model for improvement, developed by the Associates in Process Improvement (API: www.apiweb.org/) is the basis for most quality improvement techniques and is summarised in three simple questions:

What are we trying to accomplish?
How will we know that change is an improvement?
What change can we make that will result in an improvement?

How these questions are applied in practical frameworks for improvement is described in more detail below.

━━━━━━━━━━━ LEARNING ACTIVITY ━━━━━━━━━━━

Describing your aims

Think about the problem identified. Use the model for improvement to explain what you are trying to accomplish, how you will know that change is an improvement and what change can result in an improvement.

CLINICAL AUDIT

Clinical audit is a systematic activity that involves measuring performance for one or more predefined criteria, each against a standard, and repeating this until the standard is attained or until a new standard is set.

It involves stages of identifying a problem, defining criteria, setting standards for each, measuring performance and comparing this with the standard, implementing a change or changes designed to improve performance until the standard is achieved or exceeded and repeating the process, with a new standard if needed.

Identifying a problem leads to the subject for an audit, which articulates what needs to be improved and why. This is usually focused on an area where problems have been encountered in practice or it may reflect national or local guidelines where there is definitive or new evidence about effective clinical practice.

Defining criteria and setting standards is the next step. Audit criteria are explicit statements that define what elements of care are being measured (e.g. 'patients with heart attack should have a care bundle delivered by ambulance staff'). The standard defines the level of care to be achieved for each criterion, e.g. 'the care bundle should be delivered to at least 70% of patients with suspected heart attack'. Standards are often agreed by consensus but may also be based on published evidence or previous (local, national or published) audits.

Measuring performance involves collecting essential information on the criterion and comparing this with the standard to see whether there is a gap between actual and expected performance. Next, changes are implemented to improve performance, based on a theory of what is likely to work and why. An action plan can be used to record these changes including who has agreed to do what and by when.

Finally, the measurement is repeated, completing the cycle to sustain and build on improvements. The same methods are used to ensure fair comparison with the initial measurements. The repeat measurements should demonstrate that any changes have been implemented and improvements have been made. Further changes may then be required, leading to additional re-audits.

The greatest challenge is to make necessary adjustments and re-evaluate performance – in other words to complete the cycle.

THE PLAN-DO-STUDY-ACT CYCLE

The Plan–Do–Study–Act (PDSA) cycle (Gillam and Siriwardena, 2013) is an approach to rapid experimentation designed to develop, test and implement change. The rapid, repeated small scale tests of change, carried out one after another (sequential) in one organisation, or at the same time by different organisations or organisational groups (in parallel), are designed to explore whether and to what extent the changes work, before implementing one or more of these changes on a larger scale. The PDSA cycle, as its name suggests, follows consecutive stages.

The first stage is to define the objective and plan a change or changes to achieve this ('plan'). The second stage is to carry out the plan and collect data on the effects on the criteria of interest ('do'). The third stage is to analyse data and summarise what was learned ('study'). The fourth and final stage is to plan the next cycle with necessary modifications ('act').

A plan is devised to introduce change(s) for testing, making predictions about what will happen and why based on theory, with a plan to measure the change. The who, what, when, where and data to be collected, need to be specified in advance.

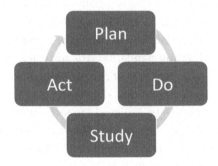

Figure 7.7   The Plan–Do–Study–Act cycle

Do(ing) involves carrying out the test by implementing the change.

Study(ing) means looking at data before and after the change, using run or control charts, usually combined with qualitative feedback to compare the data to predictions, reflecting on what was learned and summarising this.

Act(ing) entails implementing the change if it was shown to work and planning the next test, determining what modifications should be made.

PDSA is often poorly understood and applied (Taylor et al., 2014) when assessed against its key features, which include documentation, rapid repeated cycles of small-scale testing, prediction-based testing of change, and use of data over time.

━━━━━━━━ LEARNING ACTIVITY ━━━━━━━━

Trying solutions

Think about the problem identified. Design a PDSA or clinical audit to improve care.

LEAN MANAGEMENT

Lean management or Lean, was developed by Taiichi Ohno and others at Toyota in the 1930s, in the Toyota Production System for car manufacturing. It was later adopted by healthcare and is frequently defined as 'an integrated sociotechnical system whose main objective is to eliminate waste by concurrently reducing or minimizing supplier, customer, and internal variability' (Rotter et al., 2019). Lean is based on the notion of maximising value to service users while minimising waste – essentially, it is about more efficiently producing what service users need (Lean Enterprise Institute, 2015).

The Lean Enterprise Institute's five key principles of Lean focus on identifying value from a service user perspective, delineating the steps in the process and preserving those that create value ('the value stream') while eliminating those that do not, ensuring the steps in the process flow smoothly, enabling users to benefit (allowing them to 'pull value'), and repeating the cycle again until a state of perfection is reached (Moraros et al., 2016).

The introduction of Lean into healthcare has led to confusion about what exactly Lean is, as applied to this context. The lack of a consensus definition led to a systematic review designed to produce an operational definition of Lean. The authors found that Lean involves two key aspects: firstly, Lean philosophy, which includes Lean principles and continuous improvement; and secondly, Lean activities, which are a set of management practices, tools, or techniques which are used to improve care.

The operational definition specifies that, firstly, Lean philosophy is integrated into the organisation's mandate, guidelines or policies, demonstrated by evidence of Lean principles and evidence of continuous improvement; and secondly, at least one Lean activity is used, as demonstrated by evidence of either a Lean assessment activity or evidence of a Lean improvement activity.

Lean assessment activities include Value Stream Mapping (VSM visually maps critical steps in a process, describing and quantifying the essential features at each step in the flow of patients, supplies or information through the patient journey), spaghetti diagrams (plots, charts or models are a method of viewing data to visualize possible flows through systems), Rapid Process Improvement Workshops (RPIWs involve a three- to seven-day event where teams of patients, their families, staff and clinicians focus on one problem, identify the root cause, create solutions and implement the solution in the workplace), Gemba walks (the practice of managers observing, asking questions and learning from the front line to understand processes) and root cause analysis (Lawal et al., 2014).

Lean improvement activities are specific ways to reduce waste, such as '5S events', levelled production, visual management, standard work, and stop the line techniques. 5S is derived from the Japanese words *seiri, seiton, seisō, seiketsu* and *shitsuke*, which roughly translate as sort (discard anything irrelevant), sweep or straighten (organise what is left), simplify or shine (literally clean), standardise or systematise (organise and label), and sustain or self-discipline (ensure the activity is ongoing).

Levelled production is based on the idea that human beings like the stability, security and predictability of routines, that routines provide an environment in which schedules are standardised and tasks are repeated ('patterned production'), and that task repetition, assuming the task is done correctly, will naturally lead to improvement ('economies of repetition') as a result of the learning curve of practice. This involves understanding demand over a period of time, including effects of seasonality, adjusting for anticipated changes in demand, selecting a work rate to meet the need, working out the pace of work required, and ensuring you have the manpower to achieve this.

Daily visual management (DVM) is the use of easily accessible presentations to show activity, progress or outcomes which are widely used in the form of SPC and traffic light (green, red, amber) or similar display systems. Standard work is the practice of setting, communicating, following, and improving standards. 'Stop the line' techniques in industry involve enabling anyone on the production line to stop the process when a problem is observed or perceived – although this initially slows things down, it ultimately leads to more effective, efficient and safe processes and therefore improvements in production (Bell and Martinez, 2019). This is not widely used in healthcare, except perhaps in research, where studies can be halted on the basis of certain serious adverse events or unexpected interim results reviewed by a data monitoring and ethics committee.

Although Lean philosophy and activities, either alone or in combination with other approaches such as Six Sigma, have the potential for improving healthcare, recent systematic reviews show that evidence is lacking that they have actually brought about these anticipated benefits (Moraros et al., 2016).

SIX SIGMA

Six Sigma (6σ) was developed and introduced by an American engineer and executive, Bill Smith (William B. Smith, Jr), during the 1980s at the US telecommunications company Motorola, as a set of techniques and tools for process improvement. The term is derived from the standard Greek term, sigma (σ), for standard deviation, which is a measure of variation or spread from the mean in a normal distribution; Six Sigma is the goal of reducing defects or errors to less than six standard deviations, which means fewer than 3.4 defects per million (Chassin, 1998). This means fewer than 3 per million errors, adverse events, or failure to achieve a quality criterion (Chassin, 1998).

Introduced into healthcare during the 1980s, defective healthcare due to overuse, underuse or misuse usually occurs at much higher rates than this. Six Sigma involves a series of steps which are used to improve a process. They are summarised as define, measure, analyse, improve and control (DMAIC): *define* involves describing the current process, to *measure* is to collect and assess data on the existing process, to *analyse* entails identifying problems, *improve* requires planning, testing and implementing solutions, and *control* requires actions to ensure that improvements are sustained.

─── Further reading ───

Institute for Health Improvement (IHI) resources: www.ihi.org/resources/Pages/Changes/default.aspx.

Balestracci, D. (2015) *Data Sanity: A Quantum Leap to Unprecedented Results.* Englewood, CO: Medical Group Management Association.

Deming, W. E. (2000) *Out of the Crisis.* Cambridge, MA: MIT Press.

REFERENCES

Antonacci, G., Lennox, L., Barlow, J., Evans, L. and Reed, J. (2021) Process mapping in healthcare: a systematic review. *BMC Health Services Resarch,* 21: 342.

Balestracci, D. and Medical Group Management Association (2015) *Data Sanity: A Quantum Leap to Unprecedented Results.* Englewood, CO: Medical Group Management Association.

Bell, S. K. and Martinez, W. (2019) Every patient should be enabled to stop the line. *BMJ Quality and Safety,* 28: 172–6.

Bennett, B. and Provost, L. (2015) What's your theory? Driver diagram serves as tool for building and testing theories for improvement. [Online] www.apiweb.org/QP_whats-your-theory_201507.pdf. [Accessed 3 October 2022.]

Chassin, M. R. (1998) Is health care ready for Six Sigma quality? *Milbank Quarterly,* 76, 565–91, 510.

Cooper, A., Davies, F., Edwards, M., Anderson, P., Carson-Stevens, A., Cooke, M. W., Donaldson, L., Dale, J., Evans, B. A., Hibbert, P. D., Hughes, T. C., Porter, A., Rainer, T., Siriwardena, A., Snooks, H. and Edwards, A. (2019) The impact of general practitioners working in or alongside emergency departments: a rapid realist review. *BMJ Open,* 9: e024501.

Damschroder, L. J., Aron, D. C., Keith, R. E., Kirsh, S. R., Alexander, J. A. and Lowery, J. C. (2009) Fostering implementation of health services research findings into practice: a consolidated framework for advancing implementation science. *Implementation Science,* 4: 50.

Deming, W. E. (2000) *Out of the Crisis*. Cambridge, MA: MIT Press.

Donabedian, A. (1966) Evaluating the quality of medical care. *Milbank Memorial Fund Quarterly*, 44, Suppl: 166–206.

Francis, J. J., O'Connor, D. and Curran, J. (2012) Theories of behaviour change synthesised into a set of theoretical groupings: introducing a thematic series on the theoretical domains framework. *Implementation Science*, 7: 35.

Gillam, S. and Siriwardena, A. N. (2013) Frameworks for improvement: clinical audit, the plan-do-study-act cycle and significant event audit. *Quality in Primary Care*, 21: 123–30.

Johnson, M. J. and May, C. R. (2015) Promoting professional behaviour change in healthcare: what interventions work, and why? A theory-led overview of systematic reviews. *BMJ Open*, 5: e008592.

Juran, J. M. and Godfrey, A. B. (1998) *Juran's Quality Handbook*. New York: McGraw Hill.

Lawal, A. K., Rotter, T., Kinsman, L., Sari, N., Harrison, L., Jeffery, C., Kutz, M., Khan, M. F. and Flynn, R. (2014) Lean management in health care: definition, concepts, methodology and effects reported (systematic review protocol). *Systematic Reviews*, 3: 103.

Lean Enterprise Institute (2015) What is Lean? [Online]. www.lean.org. [Accessed 3 Octber 2022.]

Moraros, J., Lemstra, M. and Nwankwo, C. (2016) Lean interventions in healthcare: do they actually work? A systematic literature review. *International Journal of Quality in Health Care*, 28: 150–65.

Murray, E., Treweek, S., Pope, C., Macfarlane, A., Ballini, L., Dowrick, C., Finch, T., Kennedy, A., Mair, F., O'Donnell, C., Ong, B. N., Rapley, T., Rogers, A. and May, C. (2010) Normalisation process theory: a framework for developing, evaluating and implementing complex interventions. *BMC Medicine*, 8: 63.

Nilsen, P. (2015) Making sense of implementation theories, models and frameworks. *Implementation Science*, 10: 53.

Pawson, R. (2013) *The Science of Evaluation: A Realist Manifesto*. London, Sage.

Popper, K. R. (2002) *The Logic of Scientific Discovery*. London: Routledge.

Rogers, E. M. (2003) *Diffusion of Innovations*. New York: Simon & Schuster.

Rotter, T., Plishka, C., Lawal, A., Harrison, L., Sari, N., Goodridge, D., Flynn, R., Chan, J., Fiander, M., Poksinska, B., Willoughby, K. and Kinsman, L. (2019) What is lean management in health care? Development of an operational definition for a Cochrane Systematic Review. *Evaluation and the Health Professions*, 42: 366–90.

Siriwardena, A. N., Shaw, D., Essam, N., Togher, F. J., Davy, Z., Spaight, A., Dewey, M. and ASCQI Core Group (2014) The effect of a national quality improvement collaborative on prehospital care for acute myocardial infarction and stroke in England. *Implementation Science*, 9: 17.

Taylor, D. C. and Hamdy, H. (2013) Adult learning theories: implications for learning and teaching in medical education: AMEE Guide No. 83. *Medical Teacher*, 35: e1561–72.

Taylor, M. J., McNicholas, C., Nicolay, C., Darzi, A., Bell, D. and Reed, J. E. (2014) Systematic review of the application of the plan-do-study-act method to improve quality in healthcare. *BMJ Quality and Safety*, 23: 290–8.

Togher, F. J., Davy, Z. and Siriwardena, A. N. (2013) Patients' and ambulance service clinicians' experiences of prehospital care for acute myocardial infarction and stroke: a qualitative study. *Emergency Medicine Journal*, 30: 942–8.

Varpio, L., Paradis, E., Uijtdehaage, S. and Young, M. (2020) The distinctions between theory, theoretical framework, and conceptual framework. *Academic Medicine*, 95: 989–94.

8

WORKING WITH OTHERS

Chapter summary

This chapter explores the role of the relational in improving healthcare quality. Working with others effectively is the building block of successful quality improvement in health. Research is drawn on to illustrate the importance of staff and organisational relationships in quality improvement. Several themes related to working with others in the context of health organisations are also discussed throughout to help unpick some of the challenges and opportunities of relational facets of quality improvement.

Summary and learning points

- The role of the relational in quality improvement
- The scale of the problem
- What is organisational culture?
- How to study organisational culture?
- What constitutes good relationships in healthcare teams?
- Applying person-centred values to our work
- Improving teamwork – the evidence
- Concluding remarks

THE ROLE OF THE RELATIONAL IN QUALITY IMPROVEMENT

As explored in earlier chapters, quality improvement (QI) in health can be described as a systematic approach to enhancing patient care. It is concerned with bringing about beneficial change in quality performance in health services, systems, organisation and delivery. Due to its systematic, often process driven nature, healthcare quality improvement can be an arena filled with benchmarking, toolkits, financial appraisals and the language of managerialism. You should by now have a sense of the opportunities and limitations of standardised QI approaches, often firmly rooted in the arena of industrial manufacturing.

There is a risk that the resulting proliferation of 'quality' metrics and standardised processes can at times detract from recognising the importance of the role effective human relationships play in not only implementing but also sustaining change in healthcare. Not least during the challenging global pandemic context, increased thought and planning have been given to how we can offer relational support to one another at work, along with support for those healthcare staff working from home in line with government guidance, and creatively use online technologies to facilitate connection in lieu of physical presence.

It is therefore salient to revisit understandings of human relationships at work and the extent to which they can enable high-quality effective healthcare. We have already learned about how health organisation and quality improvement can be viewed through the systems theory lens. In other words, quality and resulting patient safety are features of the total healthcare system. Therefore, elements of the system cannot just be 'improved' in isolation, as changes in one part of the system will have effects elsewhere, influencing the function of the whole. The 'system', which in line with Ludwig von Bertalanffy's (1969) ideas is formed of interacting live components much like the biological organism, is often presented as an entity that exists independently of humans themselves. Of course, this is somewhat of an inaccuracy, given how central the human component is to the function of organisational systems. Arguably, it is not only an inextricably linked component, but one that acts as the driver of the organisational mission and agendas.

Therefore, how well people can work not only independently, but also with one another within a complex system is of crucial importance. Further, the systemic complexity itself is in part created by the nuances of human relationships. One cannot underestimate the influence of the relational, in other words the interconnectedness of two or more people, on the effectiveness of quality improvement. Within the groupings and networks of people around the delivery of healthcare, we ought to consider not only the working connections between staff, but also those with the patients, the general public and the broader external environment with which healthcare organisations interact.

THE SCALE OF THE PROBLEM

Another strong rationale for improving how we work with others is the evidence that has been gathered indicating that within the NHS as an employing organisation the climate is not always facilitative of healthy staff interaction. We also know from the perspective of the NHS that for many years there has been a growing disquiet among healthcare staff as to how enabling their working environment is and the extent to which it contributes towards undermining their mental health. Effective fulfilling relationships at work are seen to play a key role in staff retention and wellbeing in health settings and in other industries (e.g. Kansky and Diener, 2017; Scanlan et al., 2013). Evidence from the healthcare field concerns itself with the wellbeing of healthcare staff with enquiry often centred around clinician burnout and its impact on quality of care (see Linzer, 2018). My own (M. K.) interest as an executive coach and trainee psychotherapist in person-centred and experiential therapy lies in the role of the relational in enabling what Carl Rogers defined as 'self-actualisation' – our innate capacity to fulfil our full potential. In other words, my work consists of studying and teaching others how relationships can help us to thrive at work, in the healthcare sector and beyond. Data indicate that there is much need for these types of team development approaches.

The annual NHS staff survey has for several years now indicated issues with a dissatisfied demotivated workforce as well as capturing feedback around instances of bullying. Whilst surveys have their limitations around sampling and bias, as well as generalisability of findings, the 2019 survey garnered responses from 569,000 staff, a response rate of 48.5%.

The respondents expressed experiencing bullying and harassment at work:

28.5% – from patients/service users, their relatives or other members of the public
12.3% – from managers
19.0% – from other colleagues

Further, a portion of staff report experiencing stress as a result of their work, a phenomenon that has been steadily increasing since 2016:

40.3% reported feeling unwell as a result of work-related stress in the last 12 months.

Nonetheless, there are some positive findings in connection with staff relationships at work:

72.3% said they receive the respect they deserve from their colleagues.

Moreover, there was some optimism regarding relationships at work, though no doubt with room for improvement:

46.6% said relationships at work are never or rarely strained

70.9% said their immediate manager encourages them at work

(Source: www.nhsstaffsurveys.com/Page/1085/Latest-Results/NHS-Staff-Survey-Results/)

We learned from the Francis Report looking into the atrocities that took place in Mid Staffordshire NHS Foundation Trust in England (see Chapter 4) that an unfavourable and suppressive organisational culture can play a key role in the extent to which quality of care is enacted or destabilised. Indeed, recommendations from the Mid Staffordshire inquiry centred around improving organisational cultures to enable individuals to speak up freely when quality of care is subpar, upholding principles of dignified care.

WHAT IS ORGANISATIONAL CULTURE?

The culture of an organisation encapsulates the ideas, rituals, social behaviours and customs that come together to create organisational 'life'. The anthropological study of human group cultures has typically been concerned with observing how experiences became encoded through symbolism. Franz Boas (1940) wrote of the *'Kulturbrille'*, highlighting the normative assumptions we make based on cultures that we are influenced by and that we belong to.

Edgar Schein (2010), a renowned scholar of organisational culture, defined it as 'A pattern of shared basic assumptions learned by a group as it solved its problems of external adaptation and internal integration … A product of joint learning.' He visualised culture as consisting of three overarching elements – artefacts, espoused beliefs and values, and basic underlying assumptions. There are elements of organisational culture which are visible (artefacts), such as the NHS logo branding and how clinical areas are clearly definable and visible for instance. NHS-espoused values include the publicly championed belief upon which it was funded – that healthcare should be universally available to all and be free at the point of access. Lastly, there are the basic underlying assumptions, which are hidden, but which manifest themselves through artefacts and espoused values. In healthcare, these are often linked to assumptions around health and the value of human life, although the NHS, as one of the largest healthcare providers in the world, has understandably not been completely free from assumptions around commercial opportunity and conflicted views around how it should be managed and funded. These expectations can be gauged from documentary analysis of policy for instance, and board meeting minutes too – they may also have an impact on the working culture and the extent to which employees then engage with the resulting espoused values and working practices.

Indeed, there has been much uncertainty for the NHS workforce. As the NHS as a taxpayer-funded national healthcare system is at the mercy of oft-changing top-down policy mandates, this may well go some way to undermine a sense of security and confidence in one's work. As Schein argued, 'human minds need cognitive stability and any challenge of a basic assumption will release anxiety and defensiveness' (2010: 50). A study by Cortvriend (2004) investigated the impact of policy-mandated organisational restructuring on NHS staff using a case study of what was formerly known as a Primary Care Trust. Cortvriend concluded that 'Employees experienced a constant cycle of change with little time for stabilisation or adjustment, leading to negativity and lowered motivation at times' (2004: 1). External quality monitoring regimes, such as that of the Care Quality Commission, which is responsible for ensuring that healthcare providers are meeting national standards, have developed approaches to help infiltrate 'closed' and difficult cultures in services such as those for mental health and disability (Frankova, 2020), whilst at the same time being accused of creating a culture of punitive surveillance (Puntis, 2014).

Crucially, good relationships go beyond those within the organisation itself, and within a complex system such as healthcare, relationships need also to be nurtured in terms of how health services interact with their external environment and vice versa. In particular, in a public taxpayer-funded healthcare system, the influence of top-down government policy on how healthcare teams operate is wide ranging. It is naïve not to consider how continuous change mandates driven by a change in government officials can undermine employee stability and in turn their morale and their wellbeing. Therefore, there is a strong rationale for change programmes that are negotiated and co-produced locally in order to gain adequate 'buy in' from the stakeholders who matter – namely staff and patients. Stakeholder relationships will be explored later on in this chapter.

How to study organisational culture?

There exist qualitative and quantitative methods for the study of organisational culture. Qualitative approaches include:

Visiting and observing
Identifying artefacts and processes
Asking insiders why things are done that way
Identifying espoused values and asking how they are implemented
Looking for inconsistencies and enquiring about them to explore the deeper
    assumptions that may determine the observed behaviour.

Proponents of quantitative approaches argue that organisational culture can be measured and quantified using validated scales such as the Organizational Culture Inventory, Quality Improvement Implementation Survey, Hospital Culture Questionnaire and several others (see Scott et al., 2003 for a review).

There is evidence indicating that an interaction of organisational culture and quality exists. It has been argued that organisational culture provides a grounding for quality improvement (Lapiņa et al., 2015), and may render some organisations more receptive to and better able to implement QI. The impact of organisational culture on efficiency (Aktaş and Sargut, 2011) and safety improvement (Mannion and Davies, 2018) (both considered to be important elements of quality) has been studied. Further, it may be that some organisations visibly embrace QI and espouse a culture of quality, both in their artefacts and behaviours, and Rafferty and colleagues (2017) created a 'Culture of Care Barometer' to ascertain the extent of this within organisations.

However, one of the key critiques of the concept of organisational culture is that it is difficult to operationalise – in other words, can culture ever be usefully measured? And if we cannot fully grasp what a particular organisation's culture is, can we ever usefully change/manipulate culture for improved working relationships and quality? Meanwhile, nebulous concepts such as 'cultural transformation' abound in health policy rhetoric. Organisational culture itself is created slowly and evolves organically over time. Therefore, a balance needs to be sought between the desire to change culture and its preservation – a balance between continuity and renewal. Otherwise, paradoxically, enforced change may result in unintended consequences, such as uncertainty, resentment and resistance – breeding cultures that are inferior to the one that was being forcibly changed.

Nonetheless, there is a wealth of research within the business and human resource management arena which centres around how one can improve working relationships and working cultures in the context of the corporation. In order to improve culture within healthcare teams, so closely intertwined with the relational, we must first seek to understand what good relationships look like.

WHAT CONSTITUTES GOOD RELATIONSHIPS IN HEALTHCARE TEAMS?

A team is a group of people with complementary skills, usually grouped together to complete a job, task or project. A team is the result of a meshing of functions and mutual support around a goal. The 'team' is a key unit of activity within organisations with soundbites such as 'there's no "I" in team' and 'teamwork makes the dream work' suggesting that teams are non-problematic. Indeed, teamwork itself refers to the combined actions of a group, especially when efficient and effective (i.e. successful in producing a desired or intended result). 'Teaming' can also be thought of as a set of behaviours that facilitate effective team member interaction. However, as we have learned, working with others within a team can be challenging and as a result can impact on employee wellbeing and the quality of healthcare service delivery.

━━━━━━━━━━ **LEARNING ACTIVITY** ━━━━━━━━━━

Think about a time when you worked within a team. Write down what made the team effective and what didn't.

How many of the elements you wrote down can be linked back to relationships at work? Is there anything you would have done differently to improve these?

Our work evaluating Clinical Effectiveness Southwark – a quality improvement scheme in primary care in a deprived borough of South-East London providing guides and online templates for chronic disease management – found that it was the sense of 'teamness' amongst the improvement team and the collaborative inclusive relationships they formed with a range of stakeholders which enabled the programme of work to embed and gain 'buy in' locally (Ashworth et al., 2020). In this vein, Gittel and colleagues (2013) underline the importance of effective collaboration in healthcare to provide the patient with holistic care in order to best support them to achieve their goals. They explore some of the communication and cultural barriers to good relationships and propose that these deeply embedded behaviours and interaction patterns which may be specific to professional groups need to be transformed in order to improve the quality of patient care. This can be achieved over time through creating and working towards shared goals, generating co-produced knowledge and mutual respect across professional boundaries. The authors also see the potential here for enhanced relational working to improve the access to and quality of care at a scale beyond individual teams.

Further, in an earlier paper, Gittel and others (2009) argued that relationships within healthcare teams can be meaningfully coordinated by creating relational pathways of interdependent work which in turn foster high-performance healthcare systems. Indeed, Cramm and Nieboer (2012) discovered that formal relational coordination of disease-management clinicians from different disciplines improved the delivery of chronic illness care. However, whilst relational coordination is a systematic method of integrating tasks around relational touchpoints, it does not necessarily account for what constitutes personally rewarding and meaningful relationships within healthcare teams. As mentioned prevously, rewarding social relationships can be viewed as an important component of wellbeing (Kansky and Diener, 2017) and poor wellbeing at work can in turn lead to healthcare professional burnout (Hall et al., 2016). In terms of quality improvement, the detrimental impact of clinician burnout on patient safety is well documented (see Hall et al., 2016 for a review).

We know that relational competencies, such as good communication, are essential core skills that are associated with enhanced health outcomes and improved satisfaction with care (e.g. Meyer et al., 2009). In order for staff to deliver quality care, they no doubt require the necessary 'bandwidth' to withstand the demands and challenges of their working lives. There is a body of evidence from the business and management literature which indicates that employee wellbeing is upheld in workplaces where staff feel valued and work as part of cohesive teams with a shared vision and values (see Mickan and Rodger, 2000 for a review). For instance, my colleague and I are currently completing some research conducted within a large multinational corporation which demonstrates how a simple and authentic 'thank you' holds much power in nurturing our working relationships. Indeed, a quote from one of our study's participants is rather apt here: '*saying "thank you" is so powerful because it lifts up the individual and it makes him* [sic] *strive harder in his work and given tasks. Being appreciated makes an individual motivated and will create a working environment free of resentments and frustrations.*' We must, however, be mindful not to individualise the relational nor view poor relationships at work as the sole responsibility of staff. It is the 'health' of the wider organisation which has much impact on 'teamness' and cohesion – the influence factors such as a realistic workload, a well-resourced working environment, the appropriate skill mix and so forth cannot be underestimated.

Good working relationships are known to impact on several workforce factors, such as recruitment and retention, employee engagement and productivity. Recruitment and retention are important considerations for organisational development. Workforce planning – the process of analysing, forecasting and monitoring workforce supply, demand and capacity – is key to an effectively run healthcare system to ensure that it has the right number of employees with the correct skills to function and to perform. Therefore, recruiting appropriately trained staff and retaining them within the organisation is key to delivering adequately resourced services to patients. If the working cultures are not deemed to be favourable by employees, it is more likely that they will not stay in their roles in the long term (e.g. Kramer et al., 2012). This can lead to a loss in skills for the team and service, as well as a drain of organisational learning and knowledge, especially if in the instance of the NHS, the workers leave it altogether.

Recruitment and retention have posed a problem for the NHS since its inception, due to growing levels of demand, developments in treatment and changing needs, as well as the perceptions and experiences of certain career pathways. For instance, general practice (GP) in England has been affected detrimentally by these trends, impacting on quality of care. Pressures affecting GP recruitment and retention include the management of an ageing population often with multimorbid presentations, along with greater demands, with delivery being moved away from acute care into general practice to achieve cost savings, compounded by reduced numbers for primary care. Therefore, GP numbers are not keeping pace with workload demands, leading to highly pressurised working environments, compounding workforce wellbeing issues further.

Employee engagement and productivity are also influenced by how effective working relationship are. Employee engagement considers the extent to which workers are committed to their workplace's vision and values, and as a result remain motivated, with an improved sense of wellbeing. Productivity can result in part from engagement as an employee. If people believe in the vision of the organisation and this is aligned to their own values it follows that they are more likely to be productive at work, leading to efficiency gains and potentially profitability for the organisation, and the wider economic system as a whole. However, the notion of productivity as a workforce ethos has been contested, whereby productivity should not subsume considerations of staff wellbeing and person-centredness (Kordowicz, 2021).

APPLYING PERSON-CENTRED VALUES TO OUR WORK

As part of my (M.K.) present training as a person-centred and experiential psychotherapist, I am beginning to immerse myself in how the relational is understood through the lens of the discipline's founding father – Carl Rogers. It is within groups, through our relationships with others, that our identities are negotiated and formed. In large part, we make sense of our context, and as part of this we negotiate what constitutes quality improvement, through our collective realities. Rogers identified some prerequisites to an effective therapeutic alliance – one that supports the client in their journey to self-actualisation – and here it is apt to highlight two of these prerequisites as pointers towards improving our relationships at work. These are 'empathic understanding' – taking the time to listen and to seek to understand our colleagues, and 'unconditional positive regard' – the acceptance of a person within a non-judgmental space, so our colleagues can share their thoughts and feelings freely and without fear. Arguably, this is how healthcare professionals relate to their patients day in, day out. It is crucial to apply these principles towards our interactions with colleagues to create a psychologically safe space that can allow our team to flourish and in turn be able to deliver high quality of care to patients. We have seen some wonderful examples of person-centred interaction taking place with the aid of digital media, through remote team coffee breaks, writing drop ins, special interest online communities and the like. It goes without saying that exploiting the 'new normal' as a means of managerial digital surveillance of the 'performance' and outputs of health staff who can work from home will only undermine trust and relational safety.

Crucially, one cannot underestimate the time it takes to achieve engagement with quality improvement initiatives, as well as to forge effective working bonds and collaborations. Often, the quality improvement initiatives which appear to have most positive outcomes are those that are shaped within pre-existing teams with established effective working processes. For instance, through our work exploring how newly appointed Primary Care Network leaders in England (Kordowicz et al., 2022) navigated these novel organisational forms, we learned of the importance of pre-existing relationships in order to achieve a clear mandate for realising an organisational purpose. Similarly, in their study of primary care reform, Scott and Hofmeyer (2007) called for the need to recognise pre-existing networks within a change context, including understanding their roles and relational impact in order to 'establish a foundation for the diffusion of innovative practice patterns that will foster collaborative relationships and improve primary healthcare systems'.

As a final point about person-centred values as a means of improving how we work with others, relational quality improvement should not only be concerned with how relationships can improve quality, but also about recognising how the quality of relationships themselves may too need to be improved. Through a Rogerian lens, our interconnectedness with others contributes to the greater whole. Healthcare organisations sit at the interface of the individual and the society, and human existence is not possible without co-existence – something that the pandemic has made us even more acutely aware of, not least in highly individualist societies. Here evidence-based government public health interventions such as mask-wearing have been received by some as an infringement of individual liberty, rather than as a small sacrifice for the benefit of many. The unprecedented times of a global pandemic call for unity and recognising the importance of working with others and the significant role relationships play in not only upholding quality of patient care, but also in nurturing staff health. The next section of this chapter will present evidence around pragmatic approaches to improving teams and how people work within them.

IMPROVING TEAMWORK - THE EVIDENCE

Leadership is recognised as a core component of effective teamwork. Schein (2010) defined leadership 'as the source of the beliefs and values and the most central issue for leaders is to understand the deeper levels of a culture ... and to deal with the anxiety that is unleashed when those assumptions are challenged'. In this vein, the King's Fund, a prominent charity health think-tank, promotes leadership as the enabler of cultural change. It argues that

> to support staff and improve care, leadership at all levels needs to be collective, compassionate and inclusive. The emergence of sustainability and transformation partnerships and integrated care systems means that

leaders also increasingly need the relational skills to lead across systems rather than just individual institutions. (King's Fund, 2019)

Indeed, government policy (Department of Health, 2015) has recognised that nurturing effective leaders is central to cultural change and resulting improvement in quality of care, in particular in light of preventing future Mid-Staffordshire-level atrocities.

The NHS Leadership Academy is a body that designs and delivers leadership training courses, most recently in line with the NHS People Plan 2020/2021, with the strapline (an example of a Scheinian Artefact) 'developing better leaders, delivering better care'. There is overwhelming evidence in cross-disciplinary literature that good-quality tailored training helps employees develop confidence and the appropriate skills to be able to deliver their functions, in turn increasing organisational effectiveness. However, it is worth considering that the ability of leaders to lead their teams well and influence the culture of the organisation is bound by contingency (Fiedler, 1972). In other words, the context and situations which the leader comes across can influence and interact with their leadership capabilities. Further, within the healthcare sphere, attention has been paid to 'hybrid' management roles and the extent to which those with prior or parallel clinical expertise make better leaders (e.g. McGivern et al., 2015).

If we consider successful leadership as one of the factors influencing how effectively staff work with one another to improve the quality of care, we need to understand what makes good leaders. Theories of leadership abound. Some of the themes contemporary theories of effective leadership focus on include:

- Authentic leadership – that an effective leader builds honest, open relationships with others
- Compassionate leadership – highlights the role of a supportive empathetic leader, not only in the way they act towards their staff, but in how they position the values of their organisation
- Neocharismatic leadership – concerns the impact a leader's personality has on their staff and within the organisation, and the extent to which this can create transformation and innovation, including contemporary critiques of traditional approaches to the study of charismatic leadership styles
- Theories of followership – all too often leadership has been studied without due attention being given to the features and understandings of their 'followers'. Followership scholarship aims to address this gap.

Therefore, methods for improving teamwork include board level (also known as C-Suite) interventions such as executive coaching and team development, working on the assumption that effective strategic senior leadership will have 'trickle down' effects in improving the functioning of the organisation. In addition, a cohesive board where directors work well with one another, is likely to be emulated throughout the organisation, though a Korean study suggested that too cohesive a board may be detrimental to the organisation, creating narrow interests (Kim, 2005). The role of middle managers is also notable. No doubt they are crucial to effective organisational functioning – often acting as the 'go-between' between senior leadership and frontline staff. Therefore, interventions to improve how well people work together in a health organisation ought to take into account the wellbeing and upskilling of middle management.

Beyond a leadership focus, there exist numerous interventions and approaches to improving teamwork. For instance, there is a body of evidence indicating that exercises such as tailored staff training and team-building activities help strengthen a team and promote worker autonomy, as well as improving attitudes (e.g. Fapohunda, 2014; Tannenbaum et al., 1992). These types of activities are thought to contribute to team cohesion and are based on the assumption that teams are more effective when they feature greater interdependency (i.e. staff are reliant on one another's skills and labour) (Gully et al., 2002).

There is a slowly emerging body of evidence in relation to the impact of quality improvement coaching. This is a relatively new field of thought and practice, with early courses being provided by the American-based but global Institute for Healthcare Improvement. QI coaches guide quality improvement teams in achieving their goals both through the provision of improvement toolkits and solution-focused behavioural coaching support. At the time of writing, several NHS Trusts are beginning to establish their own QI coach development programmes, with some ensuring that they have sufficient capacity to assign a QI coach to each of their improvement programmes. This commitment suggests a recognition of the influence of behavioural elements on the success (or failure) of improvement projects in health.

Though this is by no means an exhaustive review of modes of improving teamwork, and readers are encouraged to pursue further reading in this area to shape their own competencies, a penultimate point of note is the notion of cultural competence and its development. We touched upon meanings surrounding culture, in particular organisational culture. Cultural competence has been defined as 'a set of congruent behaviours, attitudes and policies that come together in a system, agency or amongst professionals and enables that system, agency or those professionals to work effectively in cross-cultural situations' (Cross et al., 1989). Importantly, it has been argued that 'Those responsible for ensuring health system quality should employ measurement of both patient centeredness and cultural competence as part of the process of delivering high-quality care' (Saha et al., 2008). More so than ever, we are being called upon to recognise the importance of upholding diversity and inclusivity, and how true innovation happens only at the intersection of diverse ideas. Cultural competence training can only go so far in creating an openness in how we respond to cross-cultural situations – it is paramount that the values of equality, diversity and inclusion are frequently revisited and become truly embedded in the organisation, not only in how we work with patients, but with our colleagues.

Here, in order to bring this chapter to a close, it is apt to consider that effective teamwork is not only how people work together within an organisation, but crucially the extent to which they enable the input of the wider team – namely patients, users and stakeholders. Therefore, developing working relationships extends to those relationships which are forged externally by those within the organisation. User involvement, rooted in mental health lobby groups since the late 1960s and more recently in the John Major prime ministerial era of the Citizen's Charter, has been mentioned previously in the earlier chapter on the policy background (Chapter 4). When we consider working relationships, it is worthwhile to reflect on the level to which multiple interests and agendas are included within decision-making processes and service design. Particularly, in terms of user involvement, the extent to which this is enacted simply rhetorically as a tickbox exercise, rather than as a meaningful exercise resulting in co-design of services and interventions is an important consideration for healthcare staff and leaders. Borg and colleagues (2009) argue that the power interplay between patients and staff in mental health services needs to be considered in order to effectively facilitate non-rhetorical user involvement.

In addition, particularly within a publicly owned healthcare system, there are multiple agendas and stakeholder interests to be taken into account when planning service improvements and allocating tax-funded resource. A stakeholder can be defined as someone without whose input or 'business' an organisation would no longer exist. In terms of the NHS, this includes patients, the public, policy-makers, the government, healthcare scientists, its providers, and of course, its expert staff. Therefore, a stakeholder is someone who has an interest in that company, which may be direct or indirect, and they may have direct or indirect 'stakes' in the organisation. There are pre-existing toolkits which aid the inclusion of stakeholder agendas within programme planning through stakeholder analysis. Commonly, a stakeholder matrix can be applied, taking into account the extent to which a given party holds direct influence/power in relation to planned work and what this means for working relationships.

CONCLUDING REMARKS

This chapter has provided a tour through some of the key considerations and contemporary thinking around relationships at work within healthcare teams, and their potential impact on quality improvement. Some interventions, mostly values-based, have been proposed. The overarching aim of this chapter has been to encourage you as the reader to identify the importance of nurturing positive working relationships and recognising and upholding the humanity in our colleagues and patients through person-centred approaches. The significance of effective teamwork in quality improvement cannot be underestimated – this can make or break a programme of work.

Useful web resources

Leadership Academy - Better Leaders, Better Care, Brighter Future: www.leadershipacademy.nhs.uk/

Michael West on compassionate and inclusive leadership - The King's Fund: www.kingsfund.org.uk/audio-video/michael-west-leadership

REFERENCES

Aktaş, M. and Sargut, A. (2011) How followers' need for leadership differs according to cultural values? A theoretical framework. *Today's Review of Public Administration*, 5 (4): 195–217.

Ashworth, M., Kordowicz, M. and Fakoya, I. (2020) Clinical Effectiveness Southwark: Final evaluation report on behalf of CES and The Health Foundation.

Bertalanffy, L. von (1969) *General System Theory*. New York: George Braziller.

Boas, F. (1940) *Race, Language and Culture*. Glasgow: Good Press.

Borg, M., Karlsson, B. and Kim, H.S. (2009) User involvement in community mental health services – principles and practices. *Journal of Psychiatric and Mental Health Nursing*, 16: 285–92.

Cortvriend, P. (2004) Change management of mergers: the impact on NHS staff and their psychological contracts. *Health Services Management Research*, 17 (3): 177–87.

Cramm, J. Murray and Nieboer, A. P. (2012) Relational coordination promotes quality of chronic care delivery in Dutch disease-management programs. *Health Care Management Review*, 37 (4): 301–9.

Cross, T. L., Bazron, B. J., Dennis K. W. and Isaacs, M. R. (1989) Towards a culturally competent system of care. A monograph on effective services for minority children who are severely emotionally disturbed. A project funded by the National Institute of Mental Health, Child and Adolescent Service System Program (CASSP). Washington, DC: CASSP.

Department of Health (2015) *Culture Change in the NHS: Applying the Lessons of the Francis Inquiries*. Available at: https://assets.publishing.service.gov.uk/government/uploads/system/uploads/attachment_data/file/403010/culture-change-nhs.pdf.

Fapohunda, T. M. (2014) An exploration of the effects of work life balance on productivity. *Journal of Human Resources Management and Labor Studies*, 2 (2): 71–89.

Fiedler, F. (1972) The effects of leadership training and experience: a contingency model interpretation. *Administrative Science Quarterly*, 17 (4): 453–70.

Frankova, H. (2020) Care Quality Commission strengthens its inspection of 'closed cultures'. *Nursing and Residential Care*, 22 (3): 160–2.

Gittell, J., Godfrey, M. and Thistlethwaite, J. (2013) Interprofessional collaborative practice and relational coordination: improving healthcare through relationships. *Journal of Interprofessional Care*, 27 (3): 210–13.

Gittell, J., Seidner, R. and Wimbush, J. (2009) A relational model of how high-performance work systems work. *Organization Science*, 21 (2).

Gully, S. M., Incalcaterra, K. A., Joshi, A. and Beaubien, J. M. (2002) A meta-analysis of team-efficacy, potency, and performance: interdependence and level of analysis as moderators of observed relationships. *Journal of Applied Psychology*, 87(5): 819.

Hall, L. H., Johnson, J., Watt, I., Tsipa, A. and O'Connor, D. B. (2016) Healthcare staff wellbeing, burnout, and patient safety: a systematic review. *PloS One*, 11 (7): e0159015.

Kansky, J. and Diener, E. (2017) Benefits of well-being: health, social relationships, work, and resilience. *Journal of Positive School Psychology*, 1 (2): 129–69.

Kim, Y. (2005) Board network characteristics and firm performance in Korea. *Corporate Governance: An International Review*, 13: 800–8.

King's Fund (2019) NHS Leadership and Culture: Our Position. Available: NHS leadership and culture | The King's Fund (kingsfund.org.uk) Accessed 16.01.2023.

Kordowicz, M. (2021) The problem with productivity. In D. Wheatley, I. Hardill and S. Buglass, eds. *Handbook of Research on Remote Work and Worker Well-Being in the Post-COVID-19 Era: Impacts, Challenges, and Opportunities*. Hershey, PA: IGI Global.

Kordowicz, M., Malby, R. and Mervyn, K. (2022) Primary care networks: navigating new organisational forms. *BJGP Open*. https://doi.org/BJGPO.2021.009.

Kramer, M., Halfer, D., Maguire, P. and Schmalenberg, C. (2012) Impact of healthy work environments and multistage nurse residency programs on retention of newly licensed RNs. *Journal of Nursing Administration*, 42 (3): 148–59.

Lapiņa, I., Kairiša, I. and Aramina, D. (2015) Role of organizational culture in the quality management of university. *Procedia – Social and Behavioral Sciences*, 213: 770–4.

Linzer, M. (2018) Clinician burnout and the quality of care. *JAMA Internal Medicine*, 178(10): 1331–2.

Mannion, R. and Davies, H. Understanding organisational culture for healthcare quality improvement. *BMJ*, 2018, 363: k4907.

McGivern, G., Currie, G., Ferlie, E., Fitzgerald, L. and Waring, J. (2015) Hybrid manager–professionals' identity work: the maintenance and hybridization of medical professionalism in managerial contexts. *Public Administration*, 93: 412–32.

Meyer, E. C., Sellers, D. E., Browning, D. M., McGuffie, K., Solomon, M. Z. and Truog, R. D. (2009) Difficult conversations: improving communication skills and relational abilities in health care. *Pediatric Critical Care Medicine*, 10 (3): 352–9.

Mickan, S. and Rodger, S. (2000) Characteristics of effective teams: a literature review. *Australian Health Review*, 23: 201–8.

Puntis, J. W L. (2014) Reorganisation and culture change still needed in the Care Quality Commission. *BMJ*, 2014; 348: g1440.

Rafferty, A. M. et al. (2017). Development and testing of the 'Culture of Care Barometer' (CoCB) in healthcare organisations: a mixed methods study. *BMJ Open*. e016677.

Saha, S., Beach, M. C. and Cooper, L. A. (2008) Patient centeredness, cultural competence and healthcare quality. *Journal of the National Medical Association*, 100 (11): 1275–85.

Scanlan, J. N., Meredith, P. and Poulsen, A. A. (2013) Enhancing retention of occupational therapists working in mental health: relationships between wellbeing at work and turnover intention. *Australian Occupational Therapy Journal*, 60: 395–403.

Schein, E. H. (2010) *Organizational Culture and Leadership*, 4th ed. San Francisco, CA: Jossey-Bass.

Scott, C. and Hofmeyer, A. (2007) Networks and social capital: a relational approach to primary healthcare reform. *Health Research Policy and Systems*, 5 (9).

Scott, T., Mannion, R., Davies, H. and Marshall, M. (2003) The quantitative measurement of organizational culture in health care: a review of the available instruments. *Health Services Research*, 38 (3): 923–45.

Tannenbaum, S. I., Beard, R. L. and Salas, E. (1992) Team building and its influence on team effectiveness: an examination of conceptual and empirical developments. *Advances in Psychology*, 82: 117–53.

SECTION D

EVALUATING IMPROVEMENT

9

HOW TO EVALUATE QUALITY IMPROVEMENT?

Chapter summary

Evaluation is a vital aspect of any quality improvement initiative, however small or large, simple or complex. Evaluation needs to be designed at the outset to determine whether a quality improvement initiative has worked but also to understand how and why it has achieved its outcomes and the extent to which this can be maintained and spread.

This chapter defines what we mean by evaluation and discusses how to design an evaluation using a logic model and programme theory, as well as broader theories of implementation. It describes the various pre-experimental, experimental and quasi-experimental designs that are used for evaluation of quality improvement programmes, discusses the notion of process evaluation and embedded design and highlights the importance of economic evaluation.

Summary and learning points

- Definitions
- Logic models and programme theories
- Theory in implementation and evaluation
- Randomised controlled and cluster randomised designs

- Non-randomised experimental designs
- Non-randomised control group designs
- Statistical process control
- Interrupted time series designs
- Stepped wedge designs
- Process evaluations: nested qualitative or mixed methods
- Embedded designs
- Economic evaluation

DEFINITIONS

Evaluations of quality improvement interventions aim to assess their effectiveness (relative to a comparator), impacts (change in organisational structures, process or patient outcomes), or success (relative to goals or a logic model) (Danz et al., 2010). Quality improvement initiatives are always complex interventions consisting of multiple components and usually take place within complex systems of interacting actors and constituents (Ovretveit and Gustafson, 2002). The other important aspect of an evaluation is to understand what the intervention is, how it is implemented and received, and the context or contexts in which this occurs, rather than simply to determine whether it achieves an effect, and this requires the use of process evaluation (Hulscher et al., 2003; Moore et al., 2015). Evaluation can be done independently of the intervention or it can be embedded so that the process of improvement and evaluation can be iterative and linked, while maintaining rigor and minimising bias (Barry et al., 2018).

LOGIC MODELS AND PROGRAMME THEORIES

A logic model is a diagrammatic representation of the design of any intervention, including a quality improvement intervention. The model describes the problem, the population and priorities (or aims) of the intervention, the inputs, activities and participants, the outputs and outcomes, whether short, medium or long term, intended or unintended, positive or negative. Logic models are sometimes confusingly, referred to as programme theory diagrams because both are closely interrelated (Issen et al., 2018).

A programme theory is a detailed description about how and why the intervention could or should work and the relationship between the intervention inputs (activities and participants) and outcomes in relation to the context in which they are implemented (Reed et al., 2014). The term programme theory is part of the language of evaluation, and more recently in development of research methodology,

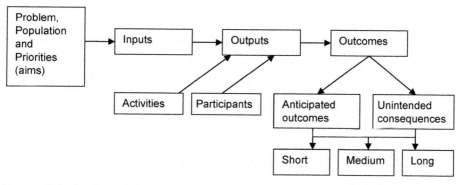

Figure 9.1 Logic model

the language of realist methods which refer to the *mechanism* by which *outcomes* are achieved in a specific *context* (Pawson and Tilley, 1997). Through the process of evaluation, the initial logic model and programme theory may be refined to describe in detail what was actually done and how it brought about any resulting change.

━━━━━━━━━━ **LEARNING ACTIVITY** ━━━━━━━━━━

Logic models and programme theories

Considering a quality improvement intervention that you have undertaken or are conducting or planning, construct a logic model and use a programme theory to describe the intervention inputs and activities and how these relate to anticipated outputs and outcomes.

THEORY IN EVALUATION

All evaluation is based on theory, whether we are aware of and acknowledge it or not. The programme theory underpinning a quality improvement can be based on a variety of implementation or intervention theories or frameworks. These can include behavioural, sociological, psychological or other broad theories and combinations of these in various theories or frameworks such as Carl May's Normalisation Process Theory (Murray et al., 2010), Louise Damschroder's Consolidated Framework for Implementation Research (Damschroder et al., 2009) or, the Promoting Action on Research Implementation in Health Services (PARIHS) framework, developed by Jo Rycroft-Malone and refined by others (Stetler et al., 2011).

Sometimes evaluators use approaches, such as realist or realistic evaluation, which develops middle range theories for how or why an intervention works and in what circumstances, referred to as context, mechanism and outcome, and use these to refine their programme theory (Pawson and Tilley, 1997). Comparative case studies are another approach that enables theory development as part of an evaluation (Yin, 2009).

RANDOMISED CONTROLLED DESIGNS

Randomised controlled trials (RCTs), when well designed and executed, are considered to be the gold standard in the traditional hierarchy of research methods. In an RCT evaluating a quality improvement intervention, the intervention is assessed against one or more comparators, assigned randomly, as one might decide on two options with the toss of a coin, although allocation is normally carried out using a computer-generated allocation and independently from knowledge of which individual or group (in a cluster randomised trial) is to be assigned to either arm, so-called allocation concealment.

RCT designs are often described in terms of the *patient* (or *population*), *intervention*, *comparator* and *outcome*, easily remembered using the acronym of PICO. One of the strengths of the RCT design is that the outcome of interest (the effect or dependent variable) can be claimed to be due to the intervention (the main cause or independent variable of interest), rather than any other feature (other independent variables) of the organisation, practitioner or patient because these alternative explanations for the outcome of interest (or confounding variables) are randomised between those receiving the intervention or the comparator. It is usual to check whether important potential confounding variables have been distributed equally, and, sometimes for key confounding variables, this is done prior to randomisation through a process called stratification.

Quality improvement interventions are always complex, that is to say, they include more than one, and usually several interacting components. Complex quality improvement interventions often involve education of members of staff, staff groups or organisational units, for example a ward, clinic or general practice. The outcomes of interest may be measured at the level of the organisational unit, particularly where this is a measure of organisational performance, or at the level of the individual patient or both. In such studies it is often not possible to randomise individual patients. This is because a person or unit that is structured or trained to behave in a particular way, cannot undo learning between patients.

Instead of randomising individual patients it is common practice to randomise a clinician or organisational unit delivering the intervention to a group or cluster of patients. In these so-called cluster randomized trials the analysis of outcomes at an individual patient level is more complicated because each individual is not entirely independent of each other because of similarities or correlation in their characteristics or attributes by virtue of attending a particular clinician, team or organisation. The degree of similarity in the outcome variable is usually described by means of the Intracluster Correlation Coefficient, between 0 (no correlation) and 1 (perfect correlation). A higher degree of correlation between patients also means cluster trials require more patients than individually randomised studies.

Bias is a systematic error introduced at any phase of research, including study design, data collection, data analysis or publication. Confounding refers to possible alternative explanations for the outcomes of a study due to a variable that influences both dependent variable and independent variable, causing a spurious and alternative explanation for an association.

In RCTs involving drug or other treatments, it is also possible to eliminate or reduce an important source of bias if the person delivering or receiving the intervention is prevented from knowing what they are giving or receiving which might affect the outcome of interest, using the technique of blinding. In a blinded trial of drugs, the treatment or comparator is disguised so that neither the patient nor the clinician knows which has been given. This is not possible in a quality improvement intervention, where it is usually obvious what is being given and received, and this may affect outcomes. This can sometimes be addressed by ensuring that the measurement of outcomes is blinded to whether the intervention or comparator was received.

The main advantage of RCTs is elimination or reduction in confounding and in some types of bias. There are important disadvantages. One disadvantage is selection bias, in that the staff or organisational units that participate in quality improvement tend to be quite different from the staff and organisational units that do not; they tend to be more enthusiastic, more open to learning, better trained, and already delivering higher quality care. This may make it more difficult to generalise the findings to the variety of contexts that occur in reality.

Another important problem is the ethical one of not delivering an intervention that is designed to improve quality of care and outcomes to those staff or units that are randomised to the comparator.

Considered from the framework of principlism, where interventions should do good (beneficence), not do harm (non-maleficence), enable choice (autonomy) and be fair (distributive justice or equity), it might be argued that those not receiving the intervention might be unfairly being denied better care without being offered a choice about what they receive. The argument for randomisation is based on the notion of equipoise, or uncertainty that the quality improvement intervention will affect outcomes positively in the way they are designed to. It is also argued that the quality improvement intervention will be spread, if it shown to be effective, and this has been successfully achieved with some quality improvement interventions, an example being PINCER, a pharmacist-led information technology intervention for medication errors (Rodgers et al., 2022).

NON-RANDOMISED EXPERIMENTAL DESIGNS

For reasons of fairness and inclusion, where equipoise is unlikely or unclear, and randomisation is therefore not possible for ethical, practical and logistical reasons, other types of designs have been used to evaluate quality improvement interventions. These include a range of uncontrolled (before-and-after), non-randomised and quasi-experimental (non-randomised control group, interrupted time series, non-randomised stepped wedge) designs.

The simplest of these is the before-and-after design, which involves introducing a quality improvement (or any other) intervention and measuring outcomes before and after its implementation. This design, also termed pre-experimental, suffers from the major weakness of not being able to account for natural variation (also termed secular trends) or other external factors affecting outcomes over time.

Natural variation means that when we measure anything at two timepoints it can either go up or down. When we look at a series of measurements over time (as in Figure 9.2) you can see that the measure goes up or down a little or a lot depending on when it is measured. This is termed natural or 'common cause' variation. If we do not know how much something is varying naturally over time, then a change can be interpreted as something getting worse or better. If an intervention is introduced and something changes, particularly for the better, then we make the mistake that it was due to our intervention, when in fact it might have happened in any case.

Although pre-experimental designs suffer from this major weakness, they can be helpful in the early stages of development of a quality improvement intervention to understand the feasibility of introducing it.

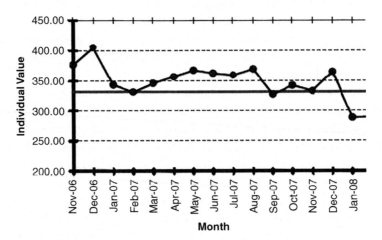

Figure 9.2   Variation over time

NON-RANDOMISED CONTROL GROUP DESIGNS

A further development from the before-and-after study is the non-randomised control group design. In this design the intervention is implemented by one or more people or sites, and a similar number of control individuals or sites are selected that are similar in all respects, except that the intervention is not introduced. Measurements are taken at baseline and following the intervention in both interventions and controls and the two are compared.

This design, although better than the simple before-and-after design, suffers from similar problems of being unable to account for secular trends in interventions or controls and alternative explanations (also termed confounding factors) for changes in either. There may also be bias in allocating interventions and controls, where intervention people or sites are more likely to effect change. Carefully selecting interventions and controls to be as closely matched for factors that might affect the outcome at the design stage may reduce the effects of confounding and these can also be accounted for in the analysis stage using statistical techniques (regression models) to account for differences found in the interventions or controls at baseline.

STATISTICAL PROCESS CONTROL

An important advance in quality improvement methods was statistical process control (SPC), a technique for analysing data over time, developed by Walter Shewhart at Bell Laboratories in the 1920s and championed by William Edwards Deming in the US and later in post-war Japan. SPC is a set of graphical and statistical techniques for understanding whether a process is in control and showing common cause (natural, random) variation or whether it is exhibiting unexpected or special cause variation (unnatural, non-random).

The two main types of graphs used to show variation over time are run charts and control charts. A control chart may be thought of as a more detailed version of a run chart, analogous to the difference between an X-ray and a CT-scan for imaging, where the latter provides a more detailed image.

In a run chart, measurements are plotted as dots with values plotted on the vertical y-axis and time plotted on the horizontal x-axis. The dots are connected by lines and a median line shows the middle value. Time intervals are usually but not necessarily equal. A minimum number, usually between 16 and 25, is needed to see if a process is stable and showing common cause variation.

The 'run' in a run chart is any sequence of dots above or below the median. A series of runs randomly distributed about the median represents common cause variation. This can be thought of as the chance of a run being above or below the median being the same as the chance of throwing heads or tails with a coin.

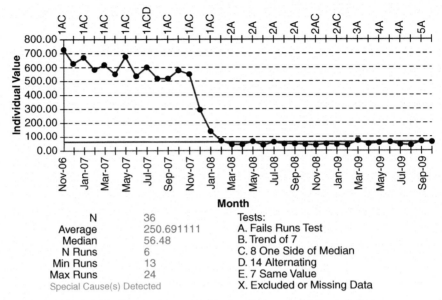

N	36	Tests:
Average	250.691111	A. Fails Runs Test
Median	56.48	B. Trend of 7
N Runs	6	C. 8 One Side of Median
Min Runs	13	D. 14 Alternating
Max Runs	24	E. 7 Same Value
Special Cause(s) Detected		X. Excluded or Missing Data

Figure 9.3   Example of special cause variation in a run chart

Three rules help to show whether there is special cause variation, and whether a change over time might be the result of an intervention. These are termed shifts, trends and runs. A shift is any sequence (or run) of at least seven dots above or below the median. A trend is a sequence of at least seven dots either increasing or decreasing (ignoring dots on the same level). Runs should be randomly distributed around the median and the right numbers of runs is calculated using a probability table.

The rules help to avoid the natural tendency for people to just look at a series of dots over time and assume there is something happening when there is not and enables a reliable and consistent interpretation of the data.

Control charts are very similar to run charts but are more sensitive for detecting significant changes over time. They have two important differences. Firstly, a mean, rather than the median, is drawn to represent the middle value. Secondly, extreme values are calculated as upper and lower control limits, depending on the type of data. For example, count data control limits are calculated based on the Poisson distribution, whereas percentage performance data are calculated using binomial distributions. Dots within the control limits represent common case variation.

The three basic rules identify the most important types of special cause variation for control charts: points outside the control limits, shifts and trends. Control charts also have a number of other rules which can be used to provide a signal that a significant change may have occurred.

So SPC using run or control charts can be used to assess change over time, and to see whether a quality improvement intervention has resulted in a change in the outcome, over and above any common cause variation, assuming that the process was stable to begin with.

INTERRUPTED TIME SERIES DESIGNS

A more detailed statistical technique to analyse change over time is the interrupted time series (ITS) design. This design analyses change of a measurement over time before or after an interruption, which is when the intervention took place.

The analysis uses segmented (or discontinuity) regression modelling to estimate the pre-intervention slope, the change in level at the intervention point, and the change in slope from pre-intervention to post-intervention. In this design the pre-intervention observation period before the intervention is introduced is acting as a control period. In addition, one or more non-intervention or control sites can be used as comparators. The technique allows stratified analyses to be conducted and confounding variables can be included in statistical models to account for differences in baseline characteristics of intervention and/or control groups. This is useful in longer-term evaluations, where it is important to take into account seasonality, and autocorrelation.

The design is very powerful for analysing change that occurs at a point in time or over a short period due to an intervention. ITS is a useful tool for quality improvement because it accounts for secular trends, can investigate outcomes with population-level data, and allows for graphical representation. Limitations of ITS include the need for a minimum number of time periods before and after an intervention to enable statistical analysis, differentiating the effects of programme components implemented together in time, and selecting suitable control populations (Penfold and Zhang, 2013).

STEPPED WEDGE DESIGNS

Stepped wedge designs are a further extension of the idea of using control periods before an intervention is introduced. These pragmatic designs require an intervention to be implemented for patients, practitioners or organisations, or groups of these, in steps at regular time intervals, so that each cluster has an initial observation or pre-intervention period and a later intervention period once the quality improvement has been introduced. Ultimately all clusters in the study will implement the intervention and together be in the intervention group. Clusters can be randomised at the start so that the intervention is implemented in a random order. Analysis of stepped wedge designs requires regression modelling, taking time into account to adjust for secular trends.

These designs are particularly useful for quality improvement interventions where for logistical, practical or financial reasons it is impossible to deliver the intervention concurrently and where it is likely that the intervention will do more good than harm, thus rendering a control arm where some do not receive the intervention unethical (Brown and Lilford, 2006).

PROCESS EVALUATIONS: NESTED QUALITATIVE OR MIXED METHODS

Quantitative and statistical analysis using the designs described above help to determine whether something has changed as a result of a quality improvement intervention. What they do not tell you is what in detail the intervention was, how and why the change occurred, and whether the same change could occur elsewhere if it was introduced in the same way. To answer these questions requires us to find out through observing or questioning those who implemented or received the intervention how and why the intervention worked in the particular context it was introduced. This requires ethnographic methods, interviews, surveys or a combination of these. Sometimes there will be different organisations or types of organisations involved in implementing the improvement, and they can form subgroups in the analysis, representing the different contexts in which the intervention may or may not succeed.

Process evaluations explore the intervention, describing it in detail and the way it was intended to achieve its effects (Hulscher et al., 2003). Quality improvement interventions are always complex, in the sense that they have more than one and usually multiple interacting components (Moore et al., 2015). They also examine what was delivered and implemented, the resources required, how delivery was achieved, how often it was delivered (dose), how close it was to what was intended (fidelity), and any changes made to it during the process of implementation. Another aspect is how the intervention actually achieves its effects or the mechanisms of impact, from the reactions and responses of those receiving the intervention, any mediators of these effects and any unintended consequences. Finally, the context in which the intervention is delivered and achieved its aims is important because this will aid understanding of whether this will work in other contexts, whether it will be maintained and the other settings to which it can be translated and spread.

Process evaluations always use qualitative methods to answer the how or why questions (O'Cathain, 2018). Sometimes they use multiple methods, combining interviews (individual or focus group) or ethnography (Vougioukalou et al., 2019) with surveys or quantitative evaluation of implementation. Qualitative and quantitative data can also be integrated in mixed methods. The different units (people, organisations) involved can be analysed separately in case study designs (Yin, 2009) and although comparative case studies have been advocated for evaluation of smaller-scale quality improvement initiatives (Harvey and Wensing, 2003), the complexity and requirements for rigour should not be underestimated.

EMBEDDED DESIGNS

Traditional evaluations have been conducted separately from quality improvement activities and by different teams (Barry et al., 2018). Although this can provide independence and reduce bias it runs the risk that the improvement cannot develop, evolve or adapt to findings from the evaluation. This idea runs counter to the notion of improvement which involves change through the use of plan–do–study–act and similar techniques designed to enhance improvement through learning.

Highly embedded designs are characterised by adaptive improvement and internal evaluation programmes which interact with each other during the process of improvement and evaluation so that both co-evolve and adapt as they learn from each other.

BOX 9.1 THE AMBULANCE HYPOS CAN STRIKE TWICE (HS2) STUDY (BOTAN ET AL., 2021)

The Ambulance Hypos can strike twice (HS2) study aimed to investigate the effect of an intervention in which ambulance personnel provided advice supported by a booklet – 'Hypos can strike twice' – issued following a hypoglycaemic event to prevent future ambulance attendances.

The study used a non-randomised stepped wedge-controlled design, where the advice booklet was introduced at different times (steps) in different areas (clusters) in the East Midlands region of the UK. During the first step (T0), no clusters were exposed to the intervention, and during the last step (T3), all clusters were exposed.

The study used a generalised linear mixed model to analyse data. This showed a reduction in the number of repeat attendances in the final step of the intervention when compared to the first (OR: 0.50, 95% CI: 0.33-0.76, p = 0.001).

A further analysis using interrupted time series design showed a significant decrease in repeat ambulance attendances for hypoglycaemia relative to the pre-intervention trend (p = 0.008). The quality of care was measured using a hypoglycaemia care bundle, which increased significantly from 63% of attendances in the period prior to the intervention to 71% of attendances during the intervention period (p <0.001).

A process evaluation using surveys and interviews of patients and clinicians found positive attitudes to the intervention from both ambulance staff and people with diabetes. Although the intervention was not always implemented, most staff members and patients found the booklet informative, easy to read and to use or explain. Patients who completed the survey reported that receiving the booklet reminded and/or encouraged them to test their blood glucose more often, adjust their diet, and have a chat/check up with their diabetes consultant.

The 'Hypos can strike twice' intervention had a positive effect on reducing repeat attendances for hypoglycaemia and achieving the care bundle, supporting the use of information booklets by ambulance clinicians to prevent future attendances for recurrent hypoglycaemic events.

━━━━━━━━━━ LEARNING ACTIVITY ━━━━━━━━━━

Designing an evaluation

Think about a quality improvement activity you are planning and decide on the possible evaluation approaches, and pros and cons of each to decide on a suitable evaluation design.

HEALTH ECONOMIC EVALUATION

One aspect of evaluation that is often overlooked is an economic evaluation. This can be a cost consequences analysis, providing a summary of costs of the quality improvement programme together with its consequences, but traditional economic evaluations involving cost-effectiveness, cost–benefit, cost–utility or cost-minimisation approaches can also be used depending on the evaluation method, costs and outcomes which are being assessed as part of the evaluation (Severens, 2003).

Further reading

Gillam, S. and Siriwardena, A. N. *Quality Improvement in Primary Care: The Essential Guide*. Boca Raton, FL: CRC Press.

Saks, M. and Allsop, J. (2019) *Researching Health: Qualitative, Quantitative and Mixed Methods*, 3rd ed. London: Sage.

Yin, R. K. (2009) *Case Study Research: Design and Methods*, 4th ed. London: Sage.

Useful web resources

Siriwardena, A. N. and Gillam, A., QI learning. http://elearning.ascqi.co.uk/. An e-learning programme designed as an introduction for health and social care professionals interested to learn more about the science and practice of quality improvement (QI).

REFERENCES

Barry, D., Kimble, L. E., Nambiar, B., Parry, G., Jha, A., Chattu, V. K., Massoud, M. R. and Goldmann, D. (2018) A framework for learning about improvement: embedded implementation and evaluation design to optimize learning. *International Journal for Quality in Health Care*, 30: 10–14.

Botan, V., Law, G. R., Laparidou, D., Rowan, E., Smith, M. D., Ridyard, C., Brewster, A., Spaight, R., Spurr, K., Mountain, P., Dunmore, S., James, J., Roberts, L., Khunti, K. and Siriwardena, A. N. (2021) The effects of a leaflet-based intervention, 'Hypos can strike twice', on recurrent hypoglycaemic attendances by ambulance services: a non-randomised stepped wedge study. *Diabetic Medicine*, 38: e14612.

Brown, C. A. and Lilford, R. J. (2006) The stepped wedge trial design: a systematic review. *BMC Medical Research Methodology*, 6: 54.

Damschroder, L. J., Aron, D. C., Keith, R. E., Kirsh, S. R., Alexander, J. A. and Lowery, J. C. (2009) Fostering implementation of health services research findings into practice: a consolidated framework for advancing implementation science. *Implementation Science*, 4: 50.

Danz, M. S., Rubenstein, L. V., Hempel, S., Foy, R., Suttorp, M., Farmer, M. M. and Shekelle, P. G. (2010) Identifying quality improvement intervention evaluations: is consensus achievable? *Quality and Safety in Health Care*, 19: 279–83.

Harvey, G. and Wensing, M. (2003) Methods for evaluation of small scale quality improvement projects. *Quality and Safety in Health Care*, 12: 210–14.

Hulscher, M. E., Laurant, M. G. and Grol, R. P. (2003) Process evaluation on quality improvement interventions. *Quality and Safety in Health Care*, 12: 40–6.

Issen, L., Woodcock, T., McNicholas, C., Lennox, L. and Reed, J. E. (2018) Criteria for evaluating programme theory diagrams in quality improvement initiatives: a structured method for appraisal. *International Journal for Quality in Health Care*, 30, 508–13.

Moore, G. F., Audrey, S., Barker, M., Bond, L., Bonell, C., Hardeman, W., Moore, L., O'Cathain, A., Tinati, T., Wight, D. and Baird, J. (2015) Process evaluation of complex interventions: Medical Research Council guidance. *BMJ*, 350: h1258.

Murray, E., Treweek, S., Pope, C., Macfarlane, A., Ballini, L., Dowrick, C., Finch, T., Kennedy, A., Mair, F., O'Donnell, C., Ong, B. N., Rapley, T., Rogers, A. and May, C. (2010) Normalisation process theory: a framework for developing, evaluating and implementing complex interventions. *BMC Medicine*, 8: 63.

O'Cathain, A. (2018) *A Practical Guide to Using Qualitative Research with Randomized Controlled Trials*. Oxford: Oxford University Press.

Ovretveit, J. and Gustafson, D. (2002) Evaluation of quality improvement programmes. *Quality and Safety in Health Care*, 11: 270–5.

Pawson, R. and Tilley, N. (1997) *Realistic Evaluation*. London: Sage.

Penfold, R. B. and Zhang, F. (2013) Use of interrupted time series analysis in evaluating health care quality improvements. *Academic Pediatrics*, 13: S38–44.

Reed, J. E., McNicholas, C., Woodcock, T., Issen, L. and Bell, D. (2014) Designing quality improvement initiatives: the action effect method, a structured approach to identifying and articulating programme theory. *BMJ Quality and Safety*, 23: 1040–8.

Rodgers, S., Taylor, A. C., Roberts, S. A., Allen, T., Ashcroft, D. M., Barrett, J., Boyd, M. J., Elliott, R. A., Khunti, K., Sheikh, A., Laparidou, D., Siriwardena, A. N., Avery, A. J. (2022) Scaling-up a pharmacist-led information technology intervention (PINCER) to reduce hazardous prescribing in general practices: multiple interrupted time series study. *PLOS Medicine* (online first DOI: 10.1371/journal.pmed.1004133).

Severens, J. L. (2003) Value for money of changing healthcare services? Economic evaluation of quality improvement. *Quality and Safety in Health Care*, 12: 366–71.

Stetler, C. B., Damschroder, L. J., Helfrich, C. D. and Hagedorn, H. J. (2011) A guide for applying a revised version of the PARIHS framework for implementation. *Implementation Science*, 6: 99.

Vougioukalou, S., Boaz, A., Gager, M. and Locock, L. (2019) The contribution of ethnography to the evaluation of quality improvement in hospital settings: reflections on observing co-design in intensive care units and lung cancer pathways in the UK. *Anthropology and Medicine*, 26: 18–32.

Yin, R. K. (2009) *Case Study Research: Design and Methods*. London: Sage.

10

SELF-EVALUATION

Chapter summary

So far, we have learned about the importance and role of evaluation in healthcare quality improvement. However, the present chapter suggests that a key element of effective quality improvement is self-evaluation – namely the act of and capacity to evaluate oneself.

Without an awareness of our strengths and gaps in skills and knowledge, it is unlikely that we will contribute at the optimal level to quality improvement. Further, given the relational aspects of quality improvement highlighted earlier in the book, having an openness and a willingness to improve the way we interact with others, is likely to be crucial in effective quality improvement. Therefore, self-evaluation can be viewed as improving qualities and the quality of the self.

To gain a deeper understanding of what constitutes self-evaluation, this chapter will unpick its various features and related terms. The second half of the chapter will present practical methods of embedding self-evaluation into quality improvement work.

Summary and learning points

- What is self-evaluation?
- Practical approaches to self-evaluation
- The self-evaluating organisation
- Critiques of self-evaluation

WHAT IS SELF-EVALUATION?

Self-evaluation can take many forms. It is often closely aligned to reflective practice, and perhaps the only distinction between the two is that self-evaluation helps to formalise the reflective process. This can be achieved by embedding self-evaluation practices into our quality improvement (QI) work, in much the same way that we have posed the argument in this book that evaluation of QI is important. Evaluation allows us to know whether what we are doing is working, if our work is improving quality for a range of patients and stakeholders, and also to identify the gaps in our practice so that we can fill them. Indeed, self-evaluation is a developmental process of reflecting on what works and what doesn't, on our learning and on the resources and skills we need in order to do better. To take this further, self-evaluation can be viewed as a QI process applied to self.

Self-evaluation is relatively well recognised in the psychotherapeutic and nursing professions and there is an established body of literature taken from these fields of clinical practice about the rationale for and methods of self-evaluation. Self-evaluation allows for the contemplation of our experiences and as the pedagogue Dewey (1938) argued 'all genuine education comes through experience'. The link between self-evaluation, learning and quality improvement has a less established evidence base, however, more formative/learning approaches to evaluation espouse some of the principles of self-evaluation, namely:

- Undertaking evaluation to promote learning
- Using feedback for continuous improvement
- Creating a culture of transparency and openness
- Promoting reflexivity – i.e. the capacity to be reflective about how our work affects us and others
- An interest in the process of improvement, not just the outcome.

The capacity for reflection is linked to learning and therefore to the extent to which we take on board development opportunities stemming from our experiences of the processes of QI design and implementation. The importance of learning from the evaluation of QI has been highlighted by Walshe and Freeman (2002). They underline the significance of understanding how and why QI interventions work, and utilising that learning for continuous development of improvement infrastructures. Further, self-reflection can be used as a pedagogical device in healthcare teaching, training and beyond, offering the student the opportunity to reflect on their own learning and areas for further improvement, in turn potentially leading to improved academic performance, although to a limited extent (Lew and Schmidt, 2011).

In nursing, self-evaluation features as part of professional training and practice. It is widely argued that nurses should become reflective practitioners (Thorpe, 2004). Self-evaluation may also be tied to the annual performance review cycle and therefore be tied to promotions and renegotiating roles and tasks, as well as future training and development opportunities. During nurse training, students may be required to self-evaluate alongside their formal assessment evaluations. The ratings provided by these two elements may not necessarily align. Interestingly, a study by Plakht and colleagues (2013) discovered that high-quality positive feedback from others is indeed associated with higher grades (more so than self-evaluation, indicating that students may under-rate themselves), whereas negative feedback is more closely aligned with self-evaluation, which too was negative and reflected in the nursing students' performance on their course. Therefore, student nurses may have a tendency to under-value their capabilities when reflecting on their performance, so ideally self-evaluation would be conducted with appropriate developmental supervision and used in combination with other performance markers, such as the feedback of colleagues, measurable outputs and outcomes, as well as patient feedback.

It is worth highlighting some of the links between the theory and practice of self-evaluation and education further. For instance, MacDonald (2005) argued for incorporating student self-evaluation of their own coursework into assessment. She states that self-reflection enables students to understand what a piece of work worthy of a higher grade than another looks like. This understanding then helps students to take on board the feedback and advice offered in order to address specific areas of weakness for improved academic performance. We can apply these understandings to the field of healthcare improvement, whereby having insights into what constitutes poor versus optimal quality of service allows improvers to effectively address gaps and opportunities.

Self-evaluation and the resulting learning can also be linked to different ways of knowing and how these are brought together to learn from our experiences. There is a plethora of quotes from humanity's greatest recorded thinkers, encouraging self-knowledge as purpose. Aristotle apparently claimed that 'knowing yourself is the beginning of all wisdom'. Kant (1965) posited, in his 1781 critique of pure reason, that 'there can be no doubt that all our knowledge begins with experience'. Feyerabend (2000) introduced the concept of 'world view' as 'a collection of beliefs, attitudes and assumptions that involves the whole person, not only the intellect, has some kind of coherence and universality, and imposes itself with a power far greater than the power of facts and fact-related theories.' We could think of the practice of self-evaluation as a means of reflecting on and learning about our world views, their roots, and their influence on our behaviours.

Additionally, the ways we come to know effect how we conceptualise our experience. We know through various modes, illustrated below, such as language, emotion, memory and so forth, and these ways of knowing are influenced by our current and developmental contexts, as well as a range of demographic and sociocultural factors. Our expectations based on prior learning therefore influence how we make sense of our experiences. Therefore, self-reflection encompasses the capacity for a 'meta-view', whereby we develop insights into the contextual and a priori determinants that affect us and our work, and in turn the process and impact of the quality improvement interventions we are stakeholders in.

Within psychotherapy, reflecting on work with clients in order to evaluate one's own 'performance' and learning within a psychotherapeutic encounter is a widely accepted and important part of training and practice. Indeed, the practice of self-evaluation and reflective writing is an important element of psychotherapy training, creating capacity for sense-making, promoting new understandings and compassion (Wright and Bolton, 2012). This allows for the therapist to evaluate their work in terms of what works and what doesn't for their client. Further, this reflective practice takes account of the socio-cultural context which surrounds and may impact on the therapeutic relationship, working on the assumption that both the therapist and client bring their own frames of reference and experiences to the session. It is therefore crucial for the therapist to nurture their awareness of how these factors may enable or limit the effectiveness of therapy (e.g. Kinsella, 2001). Indeed, evidencing self-evaluation through reflective practice is a mandatory requirement for accreditation in numerous psychotherapeutic modalities. It is worth noting that self-perception may be culturally influenced. Studies of the Dunning–Kruger effect (Dunning, 2011) (the cognitive bias identified by David Dunning and Justin Kruger) imply that those with low ability at a task will tend to overestimate their competence, and suggest that this phenomenon, identified predominantly with North American participants, may manifest differently with those from other backgrounds such as those from Japan.

To take the argument of the importance of reflecting on how the socio-cultural context influences our work and interaction with others further, and how others may be bound by theirs, more than ever are we called upon to acknowledge the impact of our work on minorities and the power asymmetries in society. Therefore, self-evaluation is also an opportunity to explore how gender and sexuality, for instance, or considerations of diversity, equality and inclusion play into how we go about our day-to-day roles. It has been argued that reflexivity enables taken-for-granted assumptions about identities, roles, perspectives, language, meanings and understandings between staff within organisations to be explored and redefined in ways that matter to the people in the workplace, which can in turn uphold diversity and inclusion (Bouten-Pinto, 2016). In their report 'Making the Difference: Diversity and Inclusion in the NHS' (2015), the health think-tank, the King's Fund, argues that diversity and inclusion are key NHS values to uphold as it seeks to eliminate discrimination against black staff and those from minorities, as well as those discriminated against due to their sexuality, religion or disability. The report claims that more inclusive teams are those that have a strong commitment to quality improvement and innovation and regularly create space to reflect on performance and seek to learn and progress. The willingness of staff to self-evaluate may be influenced by several factors such as self-awareness and insight, levels of engagement and motivation at work, stress, and so forth (Dale, 1997).

In this vein, Taylor and colleagues (1995) describe the four motives of self-evaluation, namely self-assessment, self-enhancement, self-verification and self-improvement. In order to promote self-evaluation, it is necessary that all these components are satisfied, and the authors argue for an integrative approach to self-evaluation which enables several of the four motives to be simultaneously met. It may follow that here we reflect on how health spaces and workplaces offer scope for all four, both through some formalisation such as personal development plans and revalidation self-assessment and verification exercises, but also intrinsic experiences and value alignment with self-enhancement and the extent to which the job role can contribute to this.

Moreover, one study linked self-improvement to the practice of self-compassion after making a mistake (Breines and Chen, 2012). Self-compassion is the expression of kindness towards oneself, including not responding to perceived failures with self-judgement and criticism. Instead, the authors argue that those who practise warmth and acceptance towards themselves after an error, report greater motivation to self-improvement. Therefore, one could argue, that the process of self-evaluation would be more effective and beneficial towards self-improvement if conducted with kindness and compassion to self.

Reflecting on one's work scenarios and performance can also be helpful in dealing with stress at work. In their book *Beating Stress in the NHS* (2003), Chambers and colleagues endorse the use of nurse personal development planning with a stress management focus. They suggest keeping a stress log diary, along with self-assessment scores of perceived stress, in order to evaluate stress triggers. Personal development planning for stress management is presented in the book as a holistic exercise – one in which the nurse seeks feedback from colleagues, as well as patients where appropriate. It is likely that this enables a systemic view of work stress – rather than a purely individualised one (i.e. where the burden of stress and its causal factors are firmly, and short-sightedly, placed within the remit of the nurse). Crucially, the authors then promote an action plan stemming from the self-evaluation activity, with actions linked to realistic time frames, and further evaluation of the action plan through monitoring of milestones embedded within the personal development planning. Importantly, the process of personal development planning itself has been seen as one of the means of improving clinical practice quality and developing clinical professionalism (Bossers et al., 1999).

The concept and values of medical and nursing professionalism have been widely documented. The values of clinical professionalism have been identified as:

- Integrity
- Compassion
- Altruism
- Continuous improvement
- Excellence
- Working in partnership with the wider healthcare team.

(Royal College of Pathologists, 2018)

The former editor of the *British Medical Journal*, Richard Smith, argues that professionalism is 'a key to a better healthcare system'. He refers to a 2005 Royal College of Physicians (a professional membership body with physician accreditation powers) report, entitled *Doctors in Society: Medical Professionalism in a Changing World* when supporting the notion of the doctor as a 'learner'. As outlined above, self-evaluation can be constructed as a mode of experiential or situated learning, whereby knowledge acquisition is situated in their role. In this vein, Cruess and colleagues (2006) make the connection between experiential learning through self-reflection and its role in helping to embed the values of professionalism. Indeed, Norfolk and Siriwardena (2009) developed a diagnostic tool (RDM-p) which defines, explores and explains clinical behaviour, helping to identify underperformance, whilst exploring the three core areas of relationship, diagnostics and management, underpinned by professionalism.

Lastly, a connection can be made between self-evaluation and continuous improvement. We have learned about continuous improvement total quality management approaches, but self-evaluation too can provide an on-going feedback loop to lift and maintain standards of clinical work. Therefore, self-evaluation is an important tool in developing clinical professional competency. Moreover, according to an interview study of medical educators, students and health professionals, personal awareness itself is also a key facet of professionalism (Jha et al., 2006).

PRACTICAL APPROACHES TO SELF-EVALUATION

Before reading on, have a go at the reflective activity outlined here. The prompts are designed to help you reflect on your motivations for undertaking your current work or study.

━━━━━ REFLECTIVE ACTIVITY ━━━━━

Write down what initially motivated you to do your job or undertake your course of study.

- To what extent does your current role or study meet these motivations?
- Is there anything that you can do to create greater alignment with your initial motivations?
- Is there anything that your organisation or place of study can do to create greater alignment with your initial motivations?
- What can you do with this information?

Motivations underpinning our work, or lack thereof, are important to identify as they can be good predictors of engagement with our work and levels of productivity, as well as role satisfaction. Motivated employees can also mean better organisational performance overall (e.g. Lee and Raschke, 2016). When there is a mismatch between our intrinsic (internal) motivation, such as our values, and our work, we are likely to become disengaged over time.

There are numerous frameworks and templates which can aid the process and practice of self-evaluation within the workplace. For instance, Kolb (1984) proposed that learning from experience occurs in a cyclical fashion, in what he calls an Experiential Learning Cycle. The experiential cycle is illustrated in Figure 10.1.

The cycle is concerned with the learner's cognitive (thinking) processes. He argues that effective learning takes place when a person progresses through all four elements, from a new experience or reinterpretation of existing experience, to reflecting on it, which then gives rise to a new idea or abstraction, followed by an application of those ideas to the context. Each stage is connected and supports the next. Therefore, Kolb's framework could be applied to self-evaluation, whereby as each stage is encountered it is reflected upon, driving the cycle of learning and resulting in trying out new ways of working based on experience and on reflecting on that experience.

Another notable framework for self-evaluation is Gibbs' reflective cycle. Here, six stages of exploring an experience are proposed. Its cyclical nature lends itself

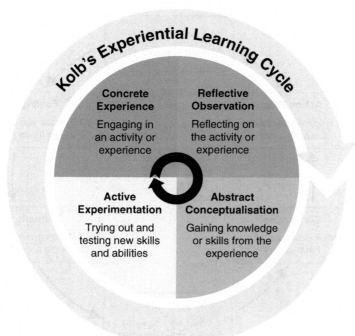

Figure 10.1   Kolb's Experiential Learning Cycle

well to continuous improvement and reflecting on repeated experiences, facilitating learning from things that went well or that need improvement. The illustration below (Figure 10.2) outlines several helpful questions to guide the health professional at each stage of the reflective process. The answers can be written down and revisited as part of self-evaluation, resulting in an action plan which then feeds into continuous reflection. The reflective cycle was proposed by Gibbs in his book *Learning by Doing* (1988); again, the focus here is on learning from experience and action in order to improve one's work and potentially one's experience of it.

Another 'well-leafed' approach to self-evaluation is the use of reflective writing and journaling about our experiences. In my own (M. K.) psychotherapy training, reflective journal entries (which are written at each training session and beyond) are a formalised requirement of the UK Council for Psychotherapy (UKCP) portfolio of learning as part of their standards of education and training. The value of reflective journaling in undergraduate nursing education for professional growth and learning – 'from practice for practice' – has also been recognised (Epp, 2008). We can also draw from the literary classic of Montaigne's 'Essays' to get a flavour of getting to know oneself through writing about experience. Michel de Montaigne (1533–1592) wrote free-ranging essays reflecting on and documenting his day-to-day life. He writes about the interdependency of his writing and experience: 'I have no more made my book than my book has made me: it is a book consubstantial with the author, of a peculiar design, a parcel of my life.' His essays represent reflections

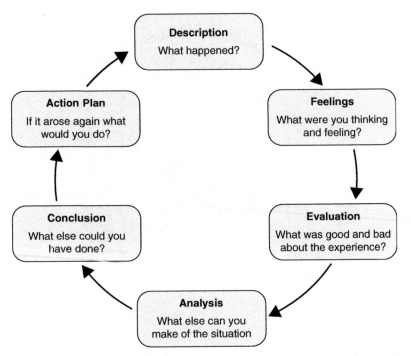

Figure 10.2   Gibbs' Reflective Cycle

upon a lifetime of learning and Montaigne remains a much-admired thinker among literary historians, having paved the way for the practice of reflective writing.

Contemporary technology can also be used to aid self-evaluation. Indeed, the COVID-19 pandemic lockdown led to growth in the use of technologies for team-working, teaching and communication. Many of the interfaces used for these reasons allow for monitoring through observation and self-observation. They also usually have a record function (where appropriate consent has been sought for this), allowing our interactions to be watched back and reflected on. Video-based self-assessment of clinical work itself has been widely used. A study by Yoo and colleagues (2009) of 40 student nurses in Korea found that video-based self-evaluation helped them develop an awareness of their strengths and areas for improvement, whilst enhancing their clinical and communication skills.

THE SELF-EVALUATING ORGANISATION

This chapter has thus far explored the theory and practice of self-evaluation from the individual perspective. However, given that quality improvement initiatives require people to work together, often at scale, it is worth asking whether self-evaluation can be enacted at the organisational level. Can self-evaluating organisations be created? Here, given the links between self-evaluation and learning, it is worth taking a look at the emergent literature regarding 'learning organisations' (a term more commonly used in the literature) to help us understand the scope for evaluation and reflection at the macro level.

One of the key influential thinkers who widely wrote about the concept of the 'learning organisation' is Peter Senge. Senge's quotes are illustrative of the culture and values that a learning organisation espouses:

> Learning organizations [are] organizations where people continually expand their capacity to create the results they truly desire, where new and expansive patterns of thinking are nurtured, where collective aspiration is set free, and where people are continually learning to see the whole together.

And:

> [The learning organisation is a place] in which you cannot not learn because learning is so insinuated into the fabric of life. (2006: 3)

To draw parallels with quality improvement, an organisation that learns is continually exploring growth and creativity according to Senge's ideas. Further, learning is embedded in the organisational culture and we can also extend this in the context of QI to learning from mistakes and failure. Sharing successes and failures has been identified as key to quality improvement efforts actually improving quality (Dixon-Woods and Martin, 2016). It is interesting here that 'doing' quality improvement is not always tantamount to improving quality. This is where evaluation as discussed in the previous chapter plays a part, as does the capacity to self-evaluate one's own role in and contributions to the programme of work.

We can draw parallels here with Edmondson and Moingeon's (1998) work, which proposes a taxonomy of organisational learning as follows: (1) residues *(organizations as residues of past learning)*; (2) communities *(organizations as collections of individuals who can learn and develop)*; (3) participation *(organizational improvement gained through intelligent activity of individual members)*; and (4) accountability *(organizational improvement gained through developing individuals' mental models)*, suggesting that there are different modes of, and perhaps levels of, organisational maturity, when it comes to their learning journeys. They also suggest that there is a distinction between organisational learning as an activity and the learning organisation as a state of being (which arguably takes time to achieve).

There are several elements to the learning organisation, including a shared vision, personal mastery, team learning, mental models and systems thinking. These were described by Senge as 'disciplines', which include micro, meso and macro levels, and typically refer to cognitions and attitudes of individuals and teams. Some benefits of embedding the disciplines of the learning organisation through eliminating the barriers to learning in health services have been documented (Vassalou, 2001). Further, the advantages of conceptualising public sector transformation as a collective learning process have been recognised, along with crucially recognising this process as one that takes time (Finger and Burgin Brand, 1999).

It may be that organisational self-evaluation can be formalised through the introduction, use and implementation of self-evaluation standards. In his paper assessing quality improvement of technical education in Saudi Arabia, Alzamil (2014) proposes that self-evaluation framework standards enable organisations to better define their aims, and to self-define the benchmarks for their performance to then work towards improving it. The author does suggest that staff within organisations may be reluctant to participate in the self-evaluation processes, lest they reveal weaknesses and underperformance. It can therefore be argued that organisational self-evaluation exercises need to be carried out in a developmental, supportive and compassionate manner, rather than as a mode of employee surveillance and control. In further support of this, Taut (2007) underlines the need for developmental contexts in order for self-evaluation to take place in organisation, especially if its resulting learning is to embed throughout. She argues that self-evaluation as a capacity-building intervention can help facilitate more accepting attitudes of participants to learning from evaluation more broadly. In a similar vein, Hardacre and Peck (2007) recognise that key features of organisational development in healthcare are activities which are 'educative, reflexive, self-examining'.

Another important element of the self-evaluating organisation is making physical and figurative space for reflection and promoting thinking time, and freeing up hectic schedules for this purpose (Prosser, 2010). Lifelong learning stemming from the institutionalisation of reflective practice has also been presented as a means of accomplishing the ideals and values of medical professionalism (Frankford et al., 2000). Here we can think of the 'Doctors' Mess' – a physical space for doctors to socialise, relax, snack and informally share and discuss clinical challenges. These areas have been removed over time from many hospitals through 'space maximisation' and cost-cutting activities, with a move by the British Medical Association to bring back on-call rooms and rest facilities, recognising their role in improving working lives and reducing clinical risk posed by tiredness (Forsythe and Suttie, 2020).

In his provocative paper at the time, entitled 'The self-evaluating organization', Wildavsky (1972) made a strong case for organisations to evaluate their own activities and the necessity of building self-awareness. He proposed a structure for evaluative activities to be incorporated into organisational life. However, he did not see this as a straightforward endeavour, arguing that there is likely a tension between day-to-day operations and the changes resulting from monitoring activities as part of evaluation, leading to resistance to organisational self-evaluation. He concluded that for self-evaluation to become truly embedded within an organisation, relational trust needs to be nurtured among social groupings within that organisation. Therefore, effective working relationships lie at the core of organisations that are self-aware and self-evaluative.

CRITIQUES OF SELF-EVALUATION

Whilst it is apparent that the benefits of self-evaluation are numerous, it is important to also reflect on the limitations and critiques of self-evaluation, and in the QI context in particular.

Self-evaluation, when formalised as part of developmental staff reviews for instance, can create a culture of reflection, transparency and learning. However, here lines can become blurred, when it becomes a part of performance monitoring and its results are used punitively, for instance through disciplinary action. Rather than leading to greater transparency, utilising formalised self-evaluation as a 'stick' rather than as a 'carrot' can undermine a culture of openness and learning from mistakes.

It could be argued that the promotion of self-evaluation practice – and potentially its proliferation through self-evaluation portfolios for the purpose of formalised professional development and accreditation – is a means of individualising practice. This means that the success and failure of a task is attributed to the individual clinician. The pitfall of this is that self-evaluation could be viewed as a means of apportioning blame to individuals and encouraging them to embody this rather than tackling systemic issues (the issues which may have contributed to the failure in the first place).

It may well be that the endorsement of reflective practice, self-evaluation, thinking time may delay day-to-day service delivery, thereby undermining quality of care. Is there a risk that there will be too much reflecting and not enough doing? Arguably, this is unlikely, as almost half of all health workers are feeling unwell because of work-related stress, according to the 2021 NHS staff survey (NHS, 2021). That is not to say that reflective spaces are the only answer. Given that nearly half of NHS workers report unsafe staffing levels (NHS, 2021), it looks as though there is a long way to go before capacity is at a level that enables downtime.

Lastly, a key critique concerns the subjective nature of self-evaluation. After all, it is a mode of expressing one's world views, reflections and providing a reflective commentary on one's experience. Self-evaluation is therefore idiographic in nature. Idiographic pertains to an individual focus, emphasising the uniqueness of personal experience. Given the range of approaches to quality improvement promoted in this book so far, it is clear that QI calls for holistic approaches, including those with a generalisable evidence base (i.e. nomothetic – the counterpart to idiographic approaches). Thus, the idiographic method of self-evaluation can be viewed as one of a complement of tools, rather than a standalone QI method.

In this chapter, we have covered the theory and practice of self-evaluation. The benefits and limitations of self-evaluation have been explored, and links made with quality improvement in health. Further, we have explored whether an organisation can also become 'self-evaluating' and how this can be enacted through organisational practices for improved quality.

Further reading

Bassot, B. (2015) *The Reflective Practice Guide: An Interdisciplinary Approach to Critical Reflection*. Abingdon: Routledge.

REFERENCES

Alzamil, Z. (2014) Quality improvement of technical education in Saudi Arabia: self-evaluation perspective. *Quality Assurance in Education*, 22 (2): 125–44.

Bossers, A., Kernaghan, J., Hodgins, L. et al. (1999) Defining and developing professionalism. *Canadian Journal of Occupational Therapy*, 66 (3): 116–21.

Bouten-Pinto, C. (2016) Reflexivity in managing diversity: a pracademic perspective. *Equality, Diversity and Inclusion*, 35 (2): 136–53.

Breines, J. G. and Chen, S. (2012). Self-compassion increases self-improvement motivation. *Personality and Social Psychology Bulletin*, 38(9), 1133–43.

Chambers R., Schwartz A. and Boath E. (2003) *Beating stress in the NHS*. Abingdon: Radcliffe Medical.

Cruess, R. et al. (2006) The professionalism mini-evaluation exercise: a preliminary investigation. *Acad Med*, 81: 74–8.

Dale, F. (1997) Stress and the personality of the psychotherapist. In V. Varma (ed.), *Stress in Psychotherapists*. London: Routledge.

Dewey, J. (1938) *Experience and Education*. New York: Collier.

Dixon-Woods, M. and Martin, G. P. (2016) Does quality improvement improve quality? *Future Hospital Journal*, 3 (3): 191–4.

Dunning, D. (2011) The Dunning–Kruger effect: on being ignorant of one's own ignorance. *Advances in Experimental Social Psychology*, 44: 247–96.

Edmondson, A. and Moingeon, B. (1998) From organizational learning to the learning organization. *Management Learning*, 29 (1): 5–20.

Epp, S. (2008) The value of reflective journaling in undergraduate nursing education: a literature review. *International Journal of Nursing Studies*, 45 (9): 1379–88.

Feyerabend, P. (2000) *Conquest of Abundance: A Tale of Abstraction Versus the Richness of Being*. Chicago: University of Chicago Press.

Finger, M. and Burgin Brand, S. (1999) The concept of the 'learning organization' applied to transformation of the public sector. In M. Easterby-Smith, L. Araujo and J. Burgoyne (1999) (eds), *Organizational Learning and the Learning Organization*. London: Sage.

Forsythe, R. O. and Suttie, S. A. (2020) Enhancing junior doctors' working lives. *Surgery (Oxford, Oxfordshire)*, 38 (10): 607–11.

Frankford, D. et al. (2000) Transforming practice organizations to foster lifelong learning commitment to medical professionalism. *Acad Med*, 75(7): 708–17.

Gibbs, G. (1988) *Learning by Doing: A Guide to Teaching and Learning Methods*. Oxford: Further Education Unit, Oxford Polytechnic.

Hardacre, J. and Peck, E. (2007) What is organisational development? In E. Peck (ed.), *Organisational Development in Healthcare: Approaches, Innovations, Achievements*. Oxford: Radcliffe.

Jha, V., Bekker, H. L., Duffy, S. R. G. and Roberts, T. E. (2006) Perceptions of professionalism in medicine: a qualitative study. *Medical Education*, 40: 1027–36.

Kant, I. (1965). *Critique of Pure Reason*. New York: St. Martin's Press.

King's Fund (2015) *Making the Difference: Diversity and Inclusion in the NHS*. Available at: www.kingsfund.org.uk/publications/making-difference-diversity-inclusion-nhs.

Kinsella, E. A. (2001) Reflections on reflective practice. *Canadian Journal of Occupational Therapy*, 68 (3): 195–8.

Kolb, D. A. (1984) Experiential *Learning: Experience as a Source of Learning and Development*. Englewood Cliffs, NJ: Prentice Hall.

Lee, M. T. and Raschke, R. L. (2016) Understanding employee motivation and organizational performance: arguments for a set-theoretic approach. *Journal of Innovation & Knowledge*, 1 (3): 162–9.

Lew, M. D. N. and Schmidt, H. G. (2011) Self-reflection and academic performance: is there a relationship? *Advances in Health Sciences Education*, 16: 529–45.

MacDonald, A. (2005) Student self-evaluation of coursework assignments: a route to a better perception of quality: case study. *Learning and Teaching in Higher Education*, 1: 102–7.

National Health Service (2021) NHS staff survey results. Accessed from: https://www.nhsstaffsurveys.com/results/ (date accessed 23.11.22)

Norfolk, T. and Siriwardena, A.N. (2009) A unifying theory of clinical practice: Relationship, Diagnostics, Management and professionalism (RDM-p). *Quality in Primary Care*, 17 (1): 37–47.

Plakht, Y., Shiyovich, A., Nusbaum, L. and Raizer, H. (2013) The association of positive and negative feedback with clinical performance, self-evaluation and practice contribution of nursing students. *Nurse Education Today*, 33 (10): 1264–8.

Prosser, S. (2010) *Effective People: Leadership and Organisation Development in Healthcare*. Oxford: Radcliffe.

Royal College of Pathologists (2018) Definition of Medical Professionalism. Available: Definition (https://www.rcpath.org/static/4738fece-a557-4d78-9bb6b58cd33ddbc5/Definition-of-medical-professionalism.pdf).

Royal College of Physicians (2005) *Doctors in Society: Medical Professionalism in a Changing World*. London: RCP.

Senge, P. (2006) *The Fifth Discipline: The Art and Practice of the Learning Organization*. London: Random House.

Taut, S. (2007) Studying self-evaluation capacity building in a large international development organization. *American Journal of Evaluation*, 28 (1): 45–59.

Taylor, S. E., Neter, E. and Wayment, H. A. (1995) Self-evaluation processes. *Personality and Social Psychology Bulletin*, 21 (12): 1278–87.

Thorpe, K. (2004) Reflective learning journals: from concept to practice. *Reflective Practice*, 5 (3): 327–43.

Vassalou, L. (2001) The learning organization in health-care services: theory and practice. *Journal of European Industrial Training*, 25 (7): 354–65.

Walshe, K. and Freeman, T. (2002) Effectiveness of quality improvement: learning from evaluations. *BMJ Quality and Safety*, 11: 85–7.

Wildavsky, A. (1972) The self-evaluating organization. *Public Administration Review*, 32 (5): 509–20.

Wright, J. and Bolton, G. (2012) *Reflective Writing in Counselling and Psychotherapy*. London: Sage.

Yoo, M. S., Son, Y. J., Kim, Y. S. and Park, J. H. (2009) Video-based self-assessment: implementation and evaluation in an undergraduate nursing course. *Nurse Education Today*, 29 (6): 585–9.

11

THE IMPORTANCE OF SUSTAINABILITY

Chapter summary

We start out with quality improvement initiatives in health with much hope for transforming the way our service is delivered. We aim for smoother processes, greater efficiency, improved morale at work and making a difference on behalf of our patients. However, the approach we undertake may be new and untested, perhaps we are applying a toolkit which worked in another context, but we have yet to learn whether it will have the same positive effects in ours. Hence, this textbook has highlighted the importance of evaluating quality improvement and reflecting on our own role within it. One of the key questions to be asked as part of the evaluation is of course 'has our quality improvement initiative worked?' It is on the basis of our answer that we then can address a further crucial question, namely 'should the quality improvement initiative be sustained?' and, if so, 'what are the implications of that?' This chapter seeks to provoke thought and provide guidance around sustainability considerations.

Summary and learning points

- What is sustainability?
- Sustainability and the resilient organisation
- How do we know when our QI programme has failed?
- Sustainability and a new dawn

WHAT IS SUSTAINABILITY?

Sustainability refers to the extent to which goods, work, activities or services are able to be sustained. It can be viewed as the process by which these items can be maintained at a certain level of functioning. Sustainability as a concept extends to environmental implications, namely the extent to which an ecological balance can be preserved, avoiding the depletion of natural resources through human production processes. Though one could argue that the corporate vs. environmental definitions are distinct, there is an important overlap that cannot be ignored. Namely, when we consider the extent to which our quality improvement (QI) initiative has worked and whether or not it should be sustained, we also need to consider its impact on quality of life and modern society, which is likely to entail considerations regarding the environmental impact of our programme of work.

In relation to environmental sustainability, many of us may recall the photography of nature thriving and air pollution levels reducing due to pandemic lockdowns, demonstrating the progress achieved by humans leading lives that interact favourably with nature. In *Forces of Reproduction: Notes for a Counter-Hegemonic Anthropocene*, Stefania Barca (2020) argues against the anthropocentric narrative which considers unrestrained production as a key enabler of human progress. 'Anthropocene' is the name given to a geological era from the commencement of human impact on the planet's ecosystems, along with climate change resulting from industrialisation. Industrialisation is tied to constructs of maleness in the literature – as a feature and extension of hegemonic masculinity and male social and economic privilege (e.g. Elliott et al., 2017). Using Audre Lorde's aphorism, Barca views the Anthropocene epoch as 'the master's house'. She proposes that 'dismantling this master's house to liberate humanity and the earth requires formidable new tools'. Therefore, a powerful significant shift is needed in our thinking and how we understand the world. Barca promotes a feminist take, one which has the capacity to bring together 'ecological, decolonial, class and species perspectives' as a way of forging alternative knowledge with which to uphold environmental justice. Perhaps we ought to pay attention to the schools of thought promoting the feminine as the cornerstone of sustainability, namely pro-environmental behaviours such as nurturance, cooperation and empathy. The potential for these traits are of course held by all genders.

Commentators have argued that sustainability is a crucial domain of quality in healthcare. Mortimer and colleagues (2018) claim that a sustainable approach contributes to the expansion of the definition of value in health, when taking into account the need to 'measure health outcomes against environmental and social impacts'. The aim of quality improvement therefore becomes enacting values of not only improving patient outcomes, but of having a positive impact on the environment and within communities. Importantly, sustainability requires a long-term view. It is not simply about utilising quality improvement to make a difference in the here and now, but it requires us to consider how our QI drives will influence our patients and society in the future.

We made the case in earlier chapters about why quality improvement matters in a time of strained resources and public health burden. Moreover, environmental challenges facing humankind provide further rationale. Notably, environmentalists and activists have urged policymakers globally to cut carbon emissions exacerbating global warming through bringing down the cost of low carbon energy and taxation, for instance. In the UK in 2021, the NHS accounted for 25% of public sector carbon dioxide emissions (King's Fund, 2012). We are also faced with plastic pollution, food and water insecurity, loss of biodiversity, deforestation and air pollution. A study by Dr Mark Ashworth from 2021 found that an increase in air pollution leads to statistically significant increases in inhaler prescriptions and respiratory consultations for children in primary care.

There is therefore a pressing case for quality improvement extending to our environmental context, along with the biopsychosocial, which can have a powerful influence on and be a causal factor in our health and wellbeing.

SUSTAINABILITY AND THE RESILIENT ORGANISATION

In the policy context chapter of this book (Chapter 4), we provided a sense of some of the political tussles that the NHS is often at the receiving end of. They can be perceived as a by-product of political short-termism – mainly springing from the desire to demonstrate having made an impact to the electorate during a four-year term to increase chances of re-election. This may, however, preclude a longer-term policy vision from taking shape. In general terms, 'longer-termism', as opposed to 'short-termism' refers to making decisions that take into account not only longer-term objectives, but also appraise the longer-term consequences. In response to the impact of the COVID-19 pandemic, The Health Foundation (an independent charity committed to improving health and healthcare in the UK), held a webinar on the subject of overcoming short-termism in health and social care policymaking. Some of the key points identified promoted creating space to solve long-term issues and drew on wide expertise, whilst opening up government departments to external challenge (The Health Foundation, 2020). Importantly, resilience planning was recognised as a consideration for future pandemic responses.

A central feature of organisational resilience is appropriate and adaptable resource and capacity. Quality improvement programmes, for instance, may have resourcing implications beyond their initial funding term. Therefore, the capacity for the sustainability of QI initiatives is a key consideration. Even successful programmes that are deemed worthy of being sustained due to having made a difference to clinical outcomes, for example, risk being discontinued if programme capacity is not in-built for longer-term success.

Organisational resilience may well be linked to having adequate resource and capacity to maintain functioning, especially within an adverse environment. There are several other elements which, according to the popular business literature, contribute to creative organisational resilience and sustainability. Responsive and skilled leadership is recognised as an important facet of sustainable organisational functioning, namely being able to understand the demands of a particular context and adapt accordingly, whilst continuing to develop and drive forward a shared vision. Leadership also influences culture and behaviours, including the extent to which an improvement culture is embedded among a team (King's Fund, 2017). Further, there needs to be an awareness of risk, and the types of events or features which can derail an improvement project. For instance, lack of senior-level 'buy-in' can undermine the impact of quality improvement work (Drew and Pandit, 2020). Importantly, the ability of an organisation to keep learning about 'what works, what doesn't and for whom' is a crucial mechanism underpinning its ability to adapt and survive.

Indeed, a learning organisation is one which is skilled at acquiring, creating and sharing knowledge, and these activities are thought to act as a catalyst for organisational quality improvement. In the spirit of a learning organisation, we can also think of capacity not only in terms of people hours, but also time to learn. Teams that are resilient are more likely to sustain their programmes of work over the long term by having a 'generalized capacity to investigate, to learn, and to act, without knowing in advance what one will be called to act upon' (Wildavsky, 1972). In terms of sustainability, the capacity of an organisation to continually learn and nurture new patterns of thinking can help it adapt effectively to changes in multifaceted internal and external conditions, significantly contributing to its survival within a shifting context.

The Program Sustainability Assessment Tool from the Center for Public Health System Science at the George Warren Brown School of Social Work is one way of assessing the sustainability of a QI programme using a ready-made toolkit. It recognises that the potential for sustainability is multifactorial. Therefore, the tool prompts us to consider and assess several domains in order to identify sustainability strengths and challenges and also guides strategic future planning for the work. The domains are as follows:

- Political support – both internal and external
- Funding stability – is there on-going funding available? Is there a favourable economic climate more broadly?
- Partnerships – including relationships with the community
- Organizational capacity – including considerations and programme integration

- Programme evaluation – along with considering how the evaluation findings have been used to engage stakeholders
- Programme adaptation – including transparency about ineffective programme components
- Communications – internal and external
- Strategic planning – through a lens of long-termism.

The tool is available here: https://cphss.wustl.edu/items/program-sustainability-assessment-tool/.

Importantly, the tool also helps to gauge the extent to which both the context and the design of the improvement programme itself is sustainable. In other words, is it likely to succeed or fail? Perhaps, only some of the elements of the QI programme warrant resourcing for their continuation. It may also be that the programme has not had the desired positive effects, failing altogether, and therefore it should not be sustained.

HOW DO WE KNOW WHEN OUR QI PROGRAMME HAS FAILED?

In order to decide whether an innovative programme of work should be sustained, we need to first understand what constitutes unsuccessful programmes and what the potential factors are which underpin their failure. Evaluation plays a crucial role here. In addition, we can draw on the literature pertaining to business innovation and learning, which holds implications for how the likelihood of failure can be decreased. First and foremost, it is worth stating that 'failure' of QI programmes may be more common than one would assume. Indeed, Davidson and others went so far as to argue that failure can be conceptualised as the 'lifeblood' of innovation in the nursing and health professions (Davidson et al., 2016).

The importance of evaluating QI, as well as evaluating our own work, has been outlined in previous chapters of this book on evaluation and self-evaluation. When considering QI programme sustainability, evaluation plays a key part. We need to know whether what we are doing is working, both to identify where to focus our QI efforts, and also to understand whether the QI interventions are having an effect. There are also several factors to consider when aiming to understand what underpins success in new programmes of work.

The chapter on troubleshooting (Chapter 7) provided the reader with several tools with which to be able to identify the potential causal mechanisms of events that go wrong. We aim to identify the root causes so that we can eliminate them to ensure the success of our project or activity. However, it may be that a single root cause is tricky to identify. The mechanisms that may lead a QI programme to be unsuccessful could be multifactorial and complex. It may be that a particular programme of work is an ill fit within a particular context or team.

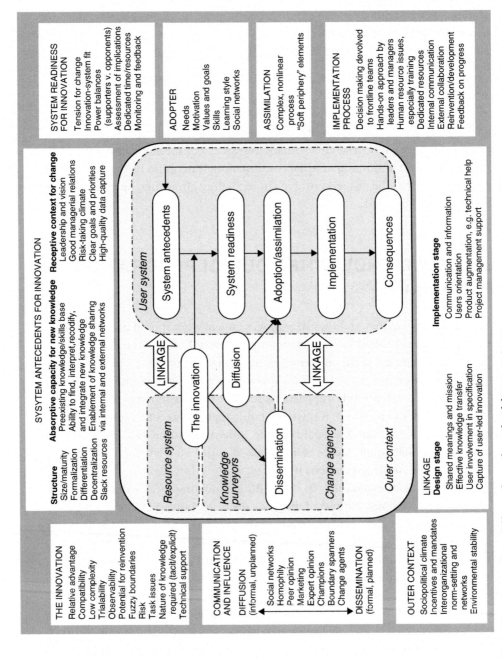

Figure 11.1   How innovation diffuses throughout healthcare systems

It is worth considering the pitfalls of improvement innovation too. For instance, by channelling resources towards quality improvement, they are taken away from other pre-established initiatives which already work well. QI and its potential for impact should be considered within the wider system in which the change is being implemented. Furthermore, Seelos and Mair (2012) argue that most value comes from perfecting routine activities so that they are done to the best possible standard, rather than through large-scale 'bells and whistles' programmes of innovation. They also argue against treating organisations as a black box, where quality improvement initiatives can be undertaken with an assumption that no confounding variables exist. Rather, organisations are formed through the complex interplay of human factors, which are often unpredictable and evolve into patterns of shared behaviour and team rituals over time.

This suggests that innovative activities such as quality improvement projects and their impacts take time to spread throughout an organisation. Everett Rogers is credited with coining the term 'diffusion of innovation'. He argues that communications play a key role in the spread of innovation, as do people. His definition of diffusion was 'the process in which an innovation is communicated through certain channels over time among the members of a social system' (Rogers, 1962). Greenhalgh and colleagues (2004) applied Rogers' ideas in their seminal paper 'Diffusion of innovations in service organizations: systematic review and recommendations'. Based on a systematic review of pre-existing studies, they proposed a conceptual model for considering the factors that play into how innovation diffuses throughout healthcare systems. The model illustrated in Figure 11.1 from this paper suggests a complex multifactorial ecosystem that the improver ought to consider when planning QI work, but also crucially when considering its potential for sustainability.

Notably, it has been argued that some failure is favourable and that the improvement drive towards ever-increasing efficiency has stifled creativity within public sector innovation. Potts (2009) promotes the concept of 'good waste' within improvement – namely, that mistakes and slack in the system are crucial in order to experiment and learn. He argues that the push for risk reduction, rather than being adaptive to and comfortable with some risk, means that creative innovative programmes of work and solutions have been suppressed within the public sector. He suggests that failure is inherent to inventiveness and experimenting with new ways of working.

━━━━━━━━━ REFLECTIVE ACTIVITY ━━━━━━━━━

Think of the activities you do throughout each week. Is there an activity you undertake regularly that you do not enjoy? Why don't you enjoy it and is it a good use of your time? Should this activity be sustained and, if not, what potentially improved way of doing things could it be replaced with?

SUSTAINABILITY AND A NEW DAWN

To draw the learning of this chapter to a close, it is worth considering new thinking around sustainability of human industry. The pandemic context has called on us to reconsider our modes of living and economic activities and philosophies towards greater localism, community building and cooperative environmentally sound practices. 'Degrowth' is a philosophy and movement concerned with sustainable economies. I (M. K.) would go so far as to argue that the essence of quality improvement cannot ignore wider determinants of health and wellbeing – crucially nurturing and rebuilding environments that support human flourishing.

The degrowth movement advocates for the creation of societies that uphold social and ecological values and sustainability. Degrowth challenges the assumption that financial profits and economic growth are testament to human progress. Rather, it promotes indicators of human prosperity, such as localism, resource sharing and happiness, over gross domestic product. Degrowth also considers the need for contemplative practices and counters fast-paced 'throwaway' goods production and short-termist productivity. In this vein, as mentioned previously, quality improvement initiatives ought to consider their long-term impacts and sustainability beyond a fast turnaround of process-driven changes.

Through my academic work, I (M. K.) conceptualise contemplation, slow-living and self-compassion as the powerful antitheses to short-termist productivity. Promoting space for rest and reflection is of utmost importance. In her article on contemplation and organization studies, Bartunek (2019) focuses on academic work, and how pressures to quantify research impact undermine the contemplative activities so necessary for knowledge generation. Indeed, Ratle and others (2020) argue for the benefits in early career academics learning how to collectively resist 'mechanisms of micro-terror' – i.e. neoliberal metricisation of performance. Bartunek also links contemplation as a means of practising compassion to self and others. No doubt these are crucial skills not only for academics like myself, but also for quality improvers. Compassion is the term given to our expressions of empathy and concern for all sentient beings, along with a will to reduce the suffering of others. Compassion and care are presented by Bartunek as key features of contemplation, as through contemplation we develop the capacity to experience life and connect with all its facets in rich depth. A key example of the practice of contemplation embedded into the work sphere is 'The Pause' – a pause at the bedside of a patient after their death, honouring their life and allowing for personal reflection through silence. This organizational intervention has been described by Ducar and Cunningham (2018) as not only a way for clinicians to regain a sense of meaning and authenticity in their work, but also as a grassroots egalitarian movement with a 'powerful systemic effect in fostering a culture of support'.

Along with a means of nurturing our desire to improve our lives and those of others, contemplative time and space can simply be a way of taking time off. Due to the pervasiveness of the productivity agenda, many of us have to relearn how to participate in downtime and may lack the ability to know when to rest and recharge (Dunn et al., 2008). Therefore, I hope that the key 'take away' from this chapter is that inherent to quality improvement sustainability is also the need for reflection and a nurturing of human values of compassion and mutual support.

In line with the degrowth philosophy, embedding the concept of sustainability as part of quality improvement 'provides a practical way for healthcare professionals to respond to ethical challenges such as climate change and social inequalities, to which we all contribute through our use of resources, and which present an urgent and unequal threat to vulnerable communities worldwide' (Mortimer et al., 2018).

Lastly, it is fitting to end this chapter with a quote from Michael West (2017). In order to create compassionate, sustainable health organisations of the future, we must also practise self-compassion: 'That means paying attention to ourselves, understanding the challenges we face in our work, and indeed in our lives generally. Empathising with ourselves, taking care of ourselves and then taking thoughtful, intelligent action to help ourselves in order that we can be who we can be and stay close to the core values that give our lives meaning.'

Further reading

Hickel, J. (2021) *Less Is More: How Degrowth Will Save the World*. London: Windmill Books.
West, M. (2011) *Compassionate Leadership*. London: Swirling Leaf Press.
Whyte, D. (2022) *Ecocide*. Manchester: Manchester University Press.

REFERENCES

Ashworth, M. et al. (2021). Spatio-temporal associations of air pollutant consultations, GP respiratory consultations and respiratory inhaler prescriptions: a 5-year study of primary care in the borough of Lambeth, South London. *Environmental Health*, 20(1): 54.

Barca, S. (2020) *Forces of Reproduction: Notes for a Counter-Hegemonic Anthropocene*. Cambridge: Cambridge University Press.

Bartunek, J. M. (2019) Contemplation and organization studies: why contemplative activities are so crucial for our academic lives. *Organization Studies*, 40: 1463–79.

Davidson, S., Weberg, D., Porter-O'Grady, T. and Malloch, K. (2016) *Leadership for Evidence-Based Innovation in Nursing and Health Professions*. Burlington, MA: Jones & Bartlett Learning.

Drew, J. R. and Pandit, M. (2020) Why healthcare leadership should embrace quality improvement. *BMJ*, 368: m872.

Ducar, M. and Cunningham, T, (2018). Honoring life after death: mapping the spread of the pause. *American Journal of Hospice and Palliative Medicine*, 36(5).

Dunn, L. et al. (2008) A conceptual model of medical student well-being: promoting resilience and preventing burnout. *Academic Psychiatry*, 32(1): 44–53.

Elliott, A. et al. (eds) (2017) *Climate Change and the Humanities*. London: Palgrave.

Greenhalgh, T., Robert, G., Macfarlane, F., Bate, P. and Kyriakidou, O. (2004) Diffusion of innovations in service organizations: systematic review and recommendations. *Milbank Quarterly*, 82 (4): 581–629.

King's Fund (2012) Sustainable health and social care: connecting environmental and financial performance. Available at: www.kingsfund.org.uk/publications/sustainable-health-and-social-care.

King's Fund (2017) Embedding a culture of quality improvement. Available at: www.kingsfund.org.uk/publications/embedding-culture-quality-improvement.

Mortimer, F., Isherwood, J., Wilkinson, A. and Vaux, E. (2018) Sustainability in quality improvement: redefining value. *Future Healthcare Journal*, 5 (2): 88–93.

Potts, J. (2009) The innovation deficit in public services: the curious problem of too much efficiency and not enough waste and failure. *Innovation*, 11 (1): 34–43.

Ratle, O. et al. (2020) Mechanisms of micro-terror? Early career CMS academics' experiences of 'targets and terror' in contemporary business schools. *Management Learning*, 51(4): 452–71.

Rogers, E. (1962) *Diffusion of Innovations*. New York: Simon & Schuster.

Seelos, C. and Mair, J. (2012) Innovation is not the Holy Grail. *Stanford Social Innovation Review*, 10 (4): 44–9. https://doi.org/10.48558/40Z4-0F36.

The Health Foundation (2020) Overcoming short-termism in policymaking after COVID-19. (Q&A with Jill Rutter.) Available at: www.health.org.uk/news-and-comment/newsletter-features/overcoming-short-termism-in-policymaking-after-covid-19.

West, M. (2017) Michael West: Collaborative and compassionate leadership. The King's Fund Leadership Summit. Available at: www.kingsfund.org.uk/audio-video/michael-west-collaborative-compassionate-leadership.

Wildavsky, A. (1972). The self-evaluating organization. *Public Administration Review*, 32 (5): 509–20.

Index